WOMB WELLNESS:

CONQUERING FIBROIDS FOR A HEALTHIER YOU

DR. MELISSA P. NELSON

All rights reserved. No part of this publication may be reproduced, distributed, or transmitted in any form or by any means, including photocopying, recording, or other electronic or mechanical methods, without the prior written permission of the publisher, except in the case of brief quotations embodied in critical reviews and certain other noncommercial uses permitted by copyright law.

TABLE OF CONTENTS

PREFACE

In the intricate tapestry of women's health, there exists a chapter that often goes unnoticed, yet profoundly impacts the lives of millions of individuals: the journey through womb wellness. As I embark on this exploration of a subject close to the core of femininity, I am both humbled and excited to present "Womb Wellness: Conquering Fibroids for a Healthier You."

The genesis of this book lies in the recognition that women's health is a holistic and interconnected experience. Our bodies are marvels of creation, and the intricate dance of hormones, emotions, and physical well-being plays a crucial role in shaping our daily lives. Fibroids, though common, have long lingered in the shadows of silence and misunderstanding. It is time to bring them into the light, to acknowledge their impact, and empower women to navigate their own paths to wellness.

This journey is a culmination of extensive research, personal stories, and a genuine desire to foster a community of support and understanding. Throughout these pages, you will find not only a wealth of information about fibroids and their multifaceted impact but also a compassionate guide to reclaiming control over your well-being. From the intricacies of medical knowledge to the empowering realm of self-care, "Womb Wellness" aims to be a companion for anyone navigating the often challenging terrain of fibroids.

As we delve into the pages of this book, let us embark on a shared expedition toward a healthier, more informed, and resilient version of ourselves. May the wisdom within these chapters serve as a beacon of light, dispelling myths, offering solace, and providing the tools necessary to conquer fibroids and embrace a healthier you.

With sincere dedication to the journey of womb wellness,

CHAPTER 1: INTRODUCTION

In the vast landscape of women's health, there exists a silent companion that often goes unnoticed until it begins to make its presence felt—fibroids. As we embark on this exploration of womb wellness, the personal connection to fibroids becomes a compelling narrative, weaving together the threads of shared experiences and untold stories.

Personal Connection to Fibroids

My journey into the realm of fibroids is not just a scholarly pursuit but a deeply personal one. Like countless others, I found myself navigating the complexities of a diagnosis that altered the course of my health and well-being. The discovery of fibroids was not merely a medical revelation; it was a journey of self-discovery, resilience, and the pursuit of understanding.

Within these pages, I will share the intimate details of my own encounter with fibroids—a journey marked by uncertainty, moments of strength, and the unwavering determination to regain control over my health. It is my hope that by unraveling my personal narrative, I can offer solace, inspiration, and a sense of camaraderie to those who find themselves on a similar path.

The Importance of Womb Wellness

Why dedicate an entire exploration to womb wellness? The answer lies in recognizing the profound impact the health of our womb has on our overall well-being. The womb is not merely a physical organ; it is a nexus of emotions, hormones, and vitality. Understanding and nurturing this intricate ecosystem is paramount to achieving a state of holistic health.

In a world where women's health is often compartmentalized, it is time to break down the barriers and acknowledge the interconnectedness of our bodies. Womb wellness is not a luxury; it is a fundamental right. By embracing this perspective, we empower ourselves to make informed choices, foster resilience, and reclaim agency over our health.

CHAPTER 2: UNDERSTANDING FIBROIDS

As we delve deeper into the intricate world of fibroids, it is essential to gain a comprehensive understanding of these noncancerous growths that can develop in the uterus. In this chapter, we will explore the various aspects of fibroids, ranging from their formation to their potential impact on one's health and well-being.

Defining Fibroids

Fibroids, medically known as uterine leiomyomas or myomas, are noncancerous growths that develop within the muscular walls of the uterus. These tumors consist of smooth muscle cells and fibrous connective tissue, and their size can range from small, undetectable nodules to large masses that significantly alter the shape and size of the uterus.

Characteristics of Fibroids:

Composition: Fibroids are primarily composed of muscle cells from the uterus and fibrous tissue.

Variability: They can vary in size, number, and location within the uterus, leading to diverse symptoms and outcomes.

Hormonal Influence: Hormones, particularly estrogen and progesterone, play a pivotal role in the development and growth of fibroids.

Types of Fibroids:

Fibroids are categorized based on their location within the uterus:

Subserosal Fibroids: These develop on the outer surface of the uterus and may press on surrounding organs, causing discomfort.

Submucosal Fibroids: Growing within the inner lining of the uterus, these can affect fertility and cause heavy menstrual bleeding.

Intramural Fibroids: Found within the muscular wall of the uterus, these can lead to the enlargement of the uterus and contribute to various symptoms.

Causes and Risk Factors:

While the exact cause of fibroid development remains elusive, several factors are associated with their occurrence:

Hormonal Influences: Estrogen and progesterone, hormones that regulate the menstrual cycle, seem to stimulate the growth of fibroids.

Genetic Predisposition: A family history of fibroids may increase an individual's likelihood of developing them.

Ethnicity and Age: Women of African descent are more likely to develop fibroids, and the risk tends to increase with age.

Signs and Symptoms:

Fibroids can manifest in various ways, and the severity of symptoms often depends on factors such as size and location:

Pelvic Pain: Some individuals may experience dull, aching pain or a sense of fullness in the pelvic region.

Menstrual Changes: Heavy menstrual bleeding, prolonged periods, and irregular cycles are common symptoms.

Urinary and Bowel Issues: Large fibroids can exert pressure on nearby organs, leading to frequent urination or constipation.

Diagnosis:

Accurate diagnosis is crucial for effective management:

Pelvic Examinations: Physical examinations may reveal the presence of enlarged or irregularly shaped uterus.

Imaging Studies: Ultrasounds, MRIs, or CT scans help visualize the size, number, and location of fibroids.

Treatment Options:

The approach to managing fibroids depends on the severity of symptoms, fertility considerations, and the individual's overall health:

Medications: Hormonal therapies may help regulate menstrual cycles and alleviate symptoms.

Minimally Invasive Procedures: Techniques such as uterine artery embolization or focused ultrasound surgery aim to shrink or remove fibroids.

Surgery: In cases of severe symptoms or fertility issues, surgical procedures like myomectomy or hysterectomy may be considered.

Understanding the nature of fibroids is a crucial step towards informed decision-making and effective management. By unraveling the complexities of their development and impact, individuals and healthcare providers can work collaboratively to address the unique challenges posed by fibroids in the context of reproductive health.

Different Types and Their Characteristics

Fibroids, though all originating in the uterine muscle tissue, can exhibit distinct characteristics based on their location within the uterus. Understanding the different types is essential for comprehending the diverse symptoms and potential complications associated with these noncancerous growths.

- **Subserosal Fibroids:**

Location: These fibroids develop on the outer surface of the uterus, extending outward.

Characteristics:

External Presence: As they grow outside the uterus, subserosal fibroids may exert pressure on surrounding organs, leading to discomfort or pain.

Limited Impact on Menstrual Flow: While they can cause pelvic pressure and backache, subserosal fibroids typically have a minimal effect on menstrual bleeding.

- **Submucosal Fibroids:**

Location: Growing within the inner lining of the uterus (the endometrium).

Characteristics:

Impact on Fertility: Submucosal fibroids can significantly affect fertility by distorting the uterine cavity, potentially interfering with implantation.

Heavy Menstrual Bleeding: These fibroids often contribute to heavy menstrual bleeding and prolonged periods.

Pelvic Pain: Due to their location, submucosal fibroids may cause pelvic pain or pressure.

- **Intramural Fibroids:**

Location: Found within the muscular wall of the uterus.

Characteristics:

Enlargement of the Uterus: Intramural fibroids can lead to the enlargement of the uterus, contributing to a feeling of fullness or bloating.

Menstrual Irregularities: They may cause irregular menstrual cycles, including heavy bleeding and prolonged periods.

Pressure Symptoms: Depending on their size, intramural fibroids can exert pressure on neighboring organs, resulting in urinary frequency or constipation.

- **Pedunculated Fibroids:**

Characteristics:

Attached by a Stalk: Pedunculated fibroids are attached to the uterus by a stalk, which can sometimes twist, causing severe pain.

May Extend into the Uterine Cavity: Some pedunculated fibroids extend into the uterine cavity, potentially impacting fertility and causing discomfort.

Mobile: Due to their attachment, these fibroids can be mobile within the pelvic cavity.

- **Cervical Fibroids:**

Location: These fibroids are found in the cervix, the lower part of the uterus that connects to the vagina.

Characteristics:

Impact on Menstruation: Cervical fibroids can lead to irregular menstrual cycles and heavy bleeding.

Pressure on the Bladder: Depending on their size, they may cause pressure on the bladder, resulting in urinary symptoms.

Challenges in Childbirth: Large cervical fibroids may pose challenges during childbirth, requiring careful management.

- **Interligamentous Fibroids:**

Location: These fibroids develop between the layers of broad ligaments, which support the uterus.

Characteristics:

May Attain Significant Size: Interligamentous fibroids can grow to a considerable size, causing a noticeable abdominal mass.

Potential Impact on Surrounding Organs: Depending on their size and location, these fibroids may compress nearby structures, leading to varied symptoms.

Surgical Complexity: Removal of interligamentous fibroids can be challenging due to their location.

Understanding the characteristics of different types of fibroids is crucial for both individuals and healthcare providers. This knowledge forms the basis for tailored treatment plans that consider the unique challenges posed by each type, ranging from fertility concerns to the impact on overall reproductive health.

CHAPTER 3: PREVALENCE AND RISK FACTORS

In this chapter, we explore the prevalence of fibroids and the multitude of factors that contribute to their development. Understanding the prevalence and associated risk factors is essential for both individuals and healthcare providers in identifying those at risk and implementing proactive measures.

Prevalence of Fibroids

Fibroids are a common occurrence, particularly among women of reproductive age. The prevalence of fibroids varies among different populations and ethnic groups. Studies indicate that up to 70-80% of women may develop fibroids by the age of 50, making them a prevalent health concern for a significant portion of the female population.

Risk Factors

Several factors contribute to an individual's likelihood of developing fibroids. Awareness of these risk factors is crucial for early detection and proactive management:

Hormonal Factors

Estrogen and Progesterone: The hormones estrogen and progesterone, which regulate the menstrual cycle, play a pivotal role in the development and growth of fibroids. As a result, factors that influence hormonal balance, such as early onset of menstruation and hormonal treatments, can impact fibroid formation.

Genetic Predisposition

Family History: A strong familial tendency exists, with women having a first-degree relative (mother or sister) with fibroids being at a higher risk. Genetic factors contribute to the susceptibility to fibroid development, and ongoing research aims to identify specific genetic markers associated with this condition.

Ethnicity

Racial Disparities: Fibroids exhibit notable racial disparities, with women of African descent having a higher risk of developing fibroids compared to women of other ethnic backgrounds. Additionally, the severity of symptoms and complications tends to be higher in this group.

Age

Reproductive Age: Fibroids are most commonly diagnosed during the reproductive years, typically between the ages of 30 and 40. The risk tends to decrease after menopause when hormonal fluctuations decrease.

Lifestyle Factors

Obesity: There is a correlation between obesity and an increased risk of fibroids. Adipose tissue, particularly in the abdominal area, produces additional estrogen, potentially contributing to fibroid development.

Other Factors

Dietary Patterns: Some studies suggest that dietary factors, such as a diet high in red meat and low in fruits and vegetables, may influence fibroid development.

However, further research is needed to establish definitive links.

Impact on Reproductive Health

Understanding the prevalence and risk factors for fibroids is crucial for assessing their impact on reproductive health. Fibroids can affect fertility, lead to complications during pregnancy, and influence choices related to family planning.

Exploring the Incidence of Fibroids

To gain a comprehensive understanding of fibroids, it is crucial to explore the incidence of these noncancerous growths across diverse populations and age groups. Incidence refers to the rate of new cases of a particular condition within a specified time period. In the context of fibroids, exploring their incidence sheds light on the frequency and distribution of these growths among different demographics.

Epidemiology of Fibroids:

Prevalence Across Ages: Fibroids are most commonly diagnosed during the reproductive years, with the incidence increasing with age. Women between the ages of 30 and 40 are more likely to develop fibroids, although they can occur at any age.

Reproductive Age Impact: The incidence of fibroids is notably linked to the hormonal fluctuations associated with the menstrual cycle, making them more prevalent during the reproductive years.

Demographic Variances:

Ethnic Disparities: Fibroids exhibit significant disparities among different ethnic groups. Women of African descent have a higher incidence of fibroids compared to women of other racial backgrounds. Additionally, the severity of symptoms tends to be more pronounced in this demographic.

Geographical Variances: Incidence rates may vary geographically, with studies indicating differences in fibroid prevalence between urban and rural areas.

Risk Factors and Incidence:

Hormonal Influences: Hormonal factors, particularly estrogen and progesterone, contribute to the incidence of fibroids. Conditions or treatments that disrupt hormonal balance may influence the likelihood of developing fibroids.

Genetic Predisposition: The familial tendency for fibroids suggests a genetic component influencing their incidence. Ongoing research aims to identify specific genetic markers associated with an increased risk.

Diagnostic Advancements:

Improved Detection: Advances in medical imaging techniques, such as ultrasound and MRI, contribute to more accurate and timely diagnosis. Increased awareness and accessibility to diagnostic tools have likely influenced the reported incidence of fibroids.

Lifestyle and Environmental Factors:

Obesity and Diet: Lifestyle factors, including obesity and dietary patterns, may impact the incidence of fibroids. Adipose tissue produces estrogen, potentially contributing to hormonal imbalances associated with fibroid development.

Environmental Exposures: Some studies suggest that exposure to certain environmental factors, such as endocrine-disrupting chemicals, may influence the incidence of fibroids. However, the relationship between environmental exposures and fibroid development requires further exploration.

Understanding the incidence of fibroids is crucial for healthcare professionals and policymakers to allocate resources effectively and implement targeted preventive measures.

Identifying Common Risk Factors

Understanding the risk factors associated with fibroids is paramount for early detection, proactive management, and personalized healthcare. Various factors contribute to an individual's susceptibility to developing these noncancerous growths. By identifying common risk factors, healthcare providers can tailor interventions and empower individuals to make informed decisions about their reproductive health.

1. Hormonal Influences:

Estrogen and Progesterone Levels: Elevated levels of estrogen and progesterone, hormones that regulate the menstrual cycle, are linked to an increased risk of fibroids. Factors such as early onset of menstruation and the use of hormonal contraceptives can influence hormonal balance.

Pregnancy and Hormonal Fluctuations: The hormonal fluctuations during pregnancy, particularly the surge in estrogen and progesterone, may contribute to fibroid growth. The risk may be higher in women who have had multiple pregnancies.

2. Genetic Predisposition:

Family History: A family history of fibroids is a significant risk factor. Women with a first-degree relative (mother or sister) who has had fibroids are more likely to develop them. Genetic factors contribute to the familial tendency, indicating a hereditary component.

Race and Ethnicity: There are notable racial disparities, with women of African descent having a higher risk of fibroids compared to women of other ethnic backgrounds. Genetic and environmental factors may contribute to these differences.

3. Age and Reproductive Factors:

Reproductive Age: Fibroids are more prevalent during the reproductive years, with the highest incidence occurring between the ages of 30 and 40. The risk tends to decrease after menopause when hormonal fluctuations diminish.

Early Menstruation and Late Menopause: Starting menstruation at an early age and reaching menopause at a later age increase the duration of hormonal exposure, potentially elevating the risk of fibroids.

4. Lifestyle and Environmental Factors:

Obesity: Obesity is associated with an increased risk of fibroids. Adipose tissue, particularly in the abdominal area, produces additional estrogen, creating an environment conducive to fibroid development.

Dietary Patterns: A diet high in red meat and low in fruits and vegetables may influence fibroid development. Nutritional factors play a role in hormonal balance and overall reproductive health.

5. Medical and Reproductive History:

Uterine Infections or Inflammation: Infections or inflammatory conditions affecting the uterus may contribute to fibroid development. Chronic inflammation can create an environment favorable to their growth.

Previous Uterine Surgery: Women with a history of uterine surgery, such as a myomectomy, may be at an increased risk of developing fibroids.

6. Environmental Exposures:

Endocrine-Disrupting Chemicals: Exposure to certain environmental factors, including endocrine-disrupting chemicals found in some plastics and pesticides, has been studied in relation to fibroid development. However, the direct link requires further investigation.

Identifying these common risk factors empowers both healthcare providers and individuals to take a proactive approach to fibroid management. Regular health check-ups, awareness of familial history, and lifestyle modifications can contribute to early detection and tailored interventions, promoting overall reproductive well-being.

CHAPTER 4: RECOGNISING SYMPTOMS

In this chapter, we delve into the diverse array of symptoms associated with fibroids. Recognizing these symptoms is pivotal for timely diagnosis, informed decision-making, and the effective management of fibroids. From subtle indicators to more pronounced signs, understanding the spectrum of symptoms provides individuals and healthcare professionals with valuable insights into the impact of fibroids on daily life.

- **Menstrual Irregularities**

Heavy Menstrual Bleeding: One of the hallmark symptoms, fibroids can lead to significantly increased menstrual flow, often accompanied by prolonged periods.

Menstrual Pain and Cramping: Fibroids may contribute to intensified menstrual cramps and pelvic pain.

- **Pelvic Discomfort and Pressure**

Pelvic Pain: Some individuals experience a persistent or intermittent dull ache or sharp pain in the pelvic region.

Pelvic Pressure: Large fibroids can exert pressure on surrounding organs, causing a sense of fullness or pressure in the pelvic area.

- **Urinary and Bowel Symptoms**

Frequent Urination: Fibroids, especially those pressing on the bladder, can lead to an increased urge to urinate.

Constipation: Pressure on the rectum may result in difficulty with bowel movements.

- ## Backache and Leg Pains

Backache: Fibroids can cause back pain, particularly if they exert pressure on the back or spine.

Leg Pain: Rarely, fibroids may press on nerves, causing leg pain or numbness.

- ## Abdominal Enlargement and Swelling

Enlarged Abdomen: In some cases, large fibroids can cause a noticeable enlargement of the lower abdomen.

Abdominal Swelling: Fibroids may contribute to a feeling of bloating or swelling.

- ## Impact on Fertility and Pregnancy

Difficulty Conceiving: Fibroids, depending on their size and location, can interfere with fertility by affecting the implantation of the embryo.

Recurrent Pregnancy Loss: Fibroids may contribute to recurrent miscarriages in some cases.

Complications During Pregnancy: Larger fibroids can lead to complications during pregnancy, such as breech position or increased likelihood of cesarean section.

Impact on Quality of Life

Fatigue: Excessive menstrual bleeding and chronic pain associated with fibroids can contribute to fatigue.

Emotional Impact: Dealing with the physical symptoms and potential fertility challenges may have emotional and psychological repercussions.

Asymptomatic Cases

It's important to note that not all individuals with fibroids experience noticeable symptoms. Some fibroids may remain asymptomatic and are only discovered during routine pelvic exams or imaging studies.

Recognizing these varied symptoms is crucial for seeking timely medical attention and initiating appropriate management strategies.

Physical and Emotional Indicators

Fibroids, beyond their physical manifestations, can have a profound impact on an individual's emotional well-being. Understanding both the physical and emotional indicators is crucial for a holistic approach to managing fibroids.

Physical Indicators:

- **Menstrual Changes:**

Heavy Menstrual Bleeding: Experiencing a sudden increase in menstrual flow or prolonged periods may indicate the presence of fibroids.

Menstrual Pain: Intensified menstrual cramps and pelvic pain can be physical indicators, often disrupting daily activities.

- **Pelvic Discomfort and Pressure:**

Pelvic Pain: Persistent or intermittent pelvic pain, ranging from dull aches to sharp discomfort, is a common physical symptom of fibroids.

Pelvic Pressure: Individuals may feel a sense of fullness or pressure in the pelvic region, especially if fibroids are large or pressing on adjacent organs.

- **Urinary and Bowel Symptoms:**

Frequent Urination: Fibroids affecting the bladder may lead to an increased urge to urinate.

Constipation: Pressure on the rectum can result in difficulty with bowel movements.

- **Backache and Leg Pains:**

Backache: Fibroids exerting pressure on the back or spine may cause back pain.

Leg Pain: Rarely, fibroids pressing on nerves can lead to leg pain or numbness.

- **Abdominal Enlargement and Swelling:**

Enlarged Abdomen: Large fibroids can cause a noticeable enlargement of the lower abdomen.

Abdominal Swelling: Fibroids may contribute to a feeling of bloating or swelling.

- **Impact on Fertility and Pregnancy**:

Difficulty Conceiving: Fibroids, especially those affecting the uterine cavity, can interfere with fertility.

Recurrent Pregnancy Loss: Fibroids may contribute to recurrent miscarriages in some cases.

Complications During Pregnancy: Larger fibroids can lead to complications during pregnancy, influencing choices such as delivery method.

Emotional Indicators:

- **Emotional Impact:**

Stress and Anxiety: Dealing with the physical symptoms, uncertainty about fertility, and potential treatment decisions can contribute to heightened stress and anxiety.

Emotional Fatigue: Coping with chronic pain and the emotional toll of managing a chronic condition may result in emotional fatigue.

- **Impact on Quality of Life:**

Fatigue: Excessive menstrual bleeding and chronic pain associated with fibroids can contribute to physical and emotional fatigue.

Concerns About Body Image: Changes in abdominal size and shape may trigger concerns about body image and self-esteem.

- **Coping Mechanisms:**

Seeking Support: Individuals may seek emotional support from friends, family, or support groups to navigate the challenges posed by fibroids.

Embracing Self-Care: Engaging in self-care practices, including relaxation techniques and activities that bring joy, can help alleviate emotional distress.

Recognizing both the physical and emotional indicators of fibroids is crucial for comprehensive healthcare. A multidimensional approach, addressing both the physical symptoms and the emotional impact, ensures a more holistic and patient-centered management of fibroids.

When to Seek Medical Attention

Timely medical attention is crucial when dealing with fibroids, as it enables early diagnosis and appropriate management. Recognizing the signs that warrant medical consultation empowers individuals to take proactive steps toward their reproductive health. Here are key indicators prompting the need for medical attention:

1. Unexplained or Sudden Changes in Menstrual Patterns:

If you experience:

Significantly Increased Menstrual Flow: Persistent heavy bleeding or sudden changes in menstrual patterns could indicate the presence of fibroids.

Severe Menstrual Pain: Intense pelvic pain or cramping during menstruation that hinders daily activities requires evaluation.

2. Pelvic Pain or Discomfort:

Seek medical attention if you have:

Persistent Pelvic Pain: Continuous or recurrent pelvic pain, irrespective of the menstrual cycle, warrants investigation.

Pelvic Pressure: A constant feeling of fullness or pressure in the pelvic region may indicate the presence of fibroids.

3. Urinary or Bowel Changes:

Consult a healthcare professional if you experience:

Frequent Urination: An increased urge to urinate, especially if it disrupts daily life.

Constipation: Difficulty with bowel movements that persists or is associated with other symptoms.

4. Back Pain, Leg Pain, or Abdominal Changes:

Medical attention is advisable if you have:

Persistent Backache: Chronic back pain, particularly if it coincides with other symptoms.

Leg Pain or Numbness: Unexplained leg pain or numbness, although rare, can be associated with fibroids pressing on nerves.

Noticeable Abdominal Enlargement: If you observe an unusual and unexplained enlargement of the lower abdomen.

5. Fertility Concerns:

If you are trying to conceive and experience:

Difficulty Getting Pregnant: If you've been actively trying to conceive without success, a healthcare provider can explore potential underlying causes, including fibroids.

Recurrent Pregnancy Loss: If you've had multiple miscarriages, it's essential to investigate potential factors, with fibroids being one of them.

6. Concerns About Reproductive Health:

Seek medical attention for:

Any Concerns About Reproductive Health: Whether related to fertility, menstrual health, or concerns about fibroids, consulting a healthcare professional can provide clarity.

7. Emotional Impact:

Consider seeking support if you experience:

Emotional Distress: The emotional toll of dealing with chronic symptoms, fertility concerns, or the impact on quality of life may warrant seeking emotional support.

8. Routine Check-ups and Screenings:

Regular gynecological check-ups are crucial for:

Early Detection: Asymptomatic fibroids can be detected through routine pelvic exams or imaging studies, especially if you are at a higher risk.

Remember, each individual's experience with fibroids is unique. If you notice any changes or have concerns about your reproductive health, don't hesitate to consult with a healthcare professional. Early intervention and a collaborative approach with your healthcare team contribute to effective fibroid management and overall well-being.

CHAPTER 5: DIAGNOSTIC PROCEDURES

In this chapter, we explore the diagnostic procedures employed to identify and assess fibroids. Early and accurate diagnosis is crucial for informed decision-making and effective management of these noncancerous growths. From routine examinations to advanced imaging techniques, understanding the diagnostic journey provides individuals and healthcare providers with valuable insights into the nature and characteristics of fibroids.

Clinical Assessment:

- **Medical History:**

Symptom Evaluation: A detailed history helps assess the nature and severity of symptoms, including changes in menstrual patterns, pelvic pain, and reproductive concerns.

Risk Factor Analysis: Understanding familial history, ethnic background, and other risk factors aids in determining the likelihood of fibroids.

- **Pelvic Examination:**

Physical Assessment: A pelvic exam allows healthcare providers to assess the size, shape, and condition of the uterus, detecting any abnormalities or signs of fibroids.

Imaging Studies:

- **Ultrasound:**

Transabdominal Ultrasound: This external ultrasound provides an overview of the uterus and is often the initial step in diagnosing fibroids.

Transvaginal Ultrasound: Using a probe inserted into the vagina, this method offers detailed images, especially for smaller fibroids.

- **Magnetic Resonance Imaging (MRI):**

High-Resolution Imaging: MRI provides detailed, high-resolution images, offering a comprehensive view of the uterus and fibroids.

Assessment of Surrounding Tissues: It helps evaluate the impact of fibroids on surrounding structures and aids in treatment planning.

- **Computed Tomography (CT) Scan:**

Detailed Imaging: CT scans may be used to provide detailed cross-sectional images, particularly when assessing large fibroids and their impact on adjacent structures.

Hysterosalpingography:

Contrast Imaging: This procedure involves injecting a contrast material into the uterus, allowing for X-ray visualization. It helps identify submucosal fibroids affecting the uterine cavity.

Hysteroscopy:

Direct Visualization: A thin, lighted tube (hysteroscope) is inserted through the cervix to visualize the inside of the uterus. It helps identify submucosal fibroids and other abnormalities.

Laparoscopy:

Minimally Invasive Exploration: Laparoscopy involves a small incision for inserting a camera to view the pelvic organs. It aids in assessing the size, location, and number of fibroids.

Biopsy:

Tissue Sampling: In certain cases, a biopsy may be performed to examine a small tissue sample from the uterus. While fibroids themselves are not cancerous, a biopsy can rule out other conditions.

Genetic Testing:

Identifying Predisposition: Genetic testing may be considered, especially when there's a strong family history of fibroids, to identify specific genetic markers associated with susceptibility.

Laboratory Tests:

Blood Tests: Assessing blood counts and hormone levels can provide additional information about the impact of fibroids on the body.

Collaborative Approach:

Multidisciplinary Consultation: In complex cases, a collaborative approach involving gynecologists, radiologists, and other specialists ensures a comprehensive assessment and tailored treatment plan.

Understanding the range of diagnostic procedures for fibroids empowers individuals to actively participate in their healthcare journey. The choice of diagnostic methods depends on factors such as symptoms, risk factors, and the need for detailed imaging.

Imaging Techniques for Fibroid Diagnosis

Accurate diagnosis of fibroids relies on advanced imaging techniques that provide detailed insights into the size, location, and characteristics of these noncancerous growths. Various imaging modalities offer distinct advantages, allowing healthcare providers to tailor treatment plans and address individual needs effectively.

Ultrasound:

- **Transabdominal Ultrasound:**

Overview of the Uterus: Utilizing a transducer on the abdominal surface, transabdominal ultrasound offers an initial assessment of the uterus and identifies potential abnormalities.

Initial Screening: It serves as a non-invasive and cost-effective screening tool, detecting large fibroids.

- **Transvaginal Ultrasound:**

Detailed Visualization: By inserting a transducer into the vagina, transvaginal ultrasound provides more detailed images of the uterus and smaller fibroids.

Improved Sensitivity: This method enhances sensitivity, aiding in the detection of submucosal and intramural fibroids.

Magnetic Resonance Imaging (MRI):

High-Resolution Imaging: MRI offers detailed, high-resolution images of the uterus and fibroids, aiding in accurate diagnosis.

Multiplanar Views: It provides multiplanar views, allowing healthcare providers to assess the relationship between fibroids and surrounding structures.

Tissue Characterization: MRI helps characterize the composition of fibroids, differentiating them from other uterine abnormalities.

Computed Tomography (CT) Scan:

Cross-Sectional Imaging: CT scans may be used for cross-sectional imaging, providing additional perspectives on large fibroids and their impact on adjacent structures.

Assessment of Pelvic Organs: It aids in evaluating the overall condition of pelvic organs and can be part of preoperative planning.

Hysterosalpingography:

Contrast Imaging: Hysterosalpingography involves injecting a contrast material into the uterus, facilitating X-ray visualization.

Detection of Submucosal Fibroids: This technique is particularly useful for identifying submucosal fibroids affecting the uterine cavity.

Hysteroscopy:

Direct Visualization: Hysteroscopy allows direct visualization of the uterine cavity using a thin, lighted tube.

Identification of Submucosal Fibroids: It is effective in identifying submucosal fibroids and other abnormalities within the uterine cavity.

Laparoscopy:

Minimally Invasive Exploration: Laparoscopy involves a small incision through which a camera is inserted to visualize the pelvic organs.

Assessment of Fibroid Characteristics: It aids in assessing the size, location, and number of fibroids, supporting treatment planning.

Genetic Testing:

Identification of Predisposition: Genetic testing may be considered to identify specific genetic markers associated with a predisposition to fibroids.

Family History Considerations: It can be particularly valuable when there is a strong family history of fibroids.

Laboratory Tests:

Blood Tests: Assessing blood counts and hormone levels provides additional information about the impact of fibroids on the body.

Rule Out Other Conditions: While not directly diagnostic for fibroids, blood tests can help rule out other conditions with similar symptoms.

Utilizing a combination of these imaging techniques allows healthcare providers to comprehensively assess fibroids and tailor treatment strategies. The choice of imaging modalities depends on factors such as the nature of symptoms, the size of fibroids, and the need for detailed characterization. Early and accurate diagnosis empowers individuals and their healthcare teams to make informed decisions regarding the management of fibroids.

Consultations with Healthcare Professionals

Engaging in consultations with healthcare professionals is a crucial step in the comprehensive management of fibroids. These interactions provide individuals with the opportunity to discuss symptoms, receive accurate diagnoses, and explore personalized treatment plans. Here's an overview of key aspects related to consultations with healthcare professionals for fibroids:

1. Selecting the Right Healthcare Provider:

Primary Care Physician: Initiate discussions with your primary care physician who can guide you through the initial evaluation and recommend appropriate specialists.

Gynecologist: Gynecologists specialize in women's reproductive health and are well-equipped to assess and manage fibroids.

Specialists: Depending on the complexity of your case, you may be referred to specialists such as reproductive endocrinologists, gynecologic surgeons, or interventional radiologists.

2. Preparing for the Consultation:

Medical History: Be prepared to provide a detailed medical history, including information about your menstrual cycles, family history, and any relevant symptoms.

List of Medications: Bring a list of current medications, including supplements, to ensure a comprehensive understanding of your health.

Questions and Concerns: Prepare a list of questions and concerns to discuss during the consultation. This ensures that all aspects of your condition are addressed.

3. Symptom Discussion:

Open Communication: Describe your symptoms in detail, including changes in menstrual patterns, pelvic pain, or any associated discomfort.

Impact on Quality of Life: Discuss how fibroids are affecting your daily life, including any challenges related to work, relationships, or emotional well-being.

4. Physical Examination:

Pelvic Exam: A pelvic exam may be conducted to assess the size, shape, and condition of the uterus. This helps in identifying any physical signs of fibroids.

Additional Tests: Depending on the initial assessment, healthcare providers may recommend additional tests, such as ultrasound or imaging studies, to gather more information.

5. Diagnostic Interpretation:

Review of Test Results: Healthcare professionals will interpret diagnostic test results, discussing findings related to the size, location, and characteristics of fibroids.

Discussion of Treatment Options: Based on the diagnosis, healthcare providers will discuss various treatment options, ranging from conservative management to surgical interventions.

6. Treatment Planning:

Personalized Approach: Treatment plans are tailored to individual needs, taking into account factors such as symptom severity, reproductive goals, and overall health.

Multidisciplinary Collaboration: In complex cases, healthcare providers may collaborate with specialists from different fields to ensure a comprehensive and integrated approach to care.

7. Addressing Fertility Concerns:

Fertility Evaluation: If fertility is a concern, discussions will involve evaluating the impact of fibroids on reproductive health and exploring fertility preservation options.

Reproductive Endocrinologist: For individuals seeking fertility treatments, a reproductive endocrinologist may be involved in the consultation.

8. Patient Education:

Understanding Fibroids: Healthcare providers will ensure that individuals have a clear understanding of fibroids, including their causes, potential complications, and available treatment options.

Lifestyle Recommendations: Education on lifestyle modifications, including dietary changes and stress management, may be provided to complement medical interventions.

9. Follow-Up Care:

Monitoring and Adjustments: Regular follow-up appointments allow healthcare providers to monitor the effectiveness of treatment and make any necessary adjustments to the plan.

Open Communication: Maintain open communication with your healthcare team, reporting any changes in symptoms or concerns promptly.

Engaging in consultations with healthcare professionals empowers individuals to actively participate in their fibroid management. The collaborative relationship between patients and healthcare providers ensures that treatment plans are tailored to individual needs, promoting overall well-being and reproductive health.

CHAPTER 6: TREATMENT OPTIONS

In this chapter, we explore a spectrum of treatment options for fibroids, ranging from conservative approaches to surgical interventions. The choice of treatment depends on factors such as the size and location of fibroids, severity of symptoms, and individual health goals. Understanding the available options empowers individuals to make informed decisions about their fibroid management.

Conservative Management:

- **Watchful Waiting:**

Monitoring Symptoms: In cases of asymptomatic or minimally symptomatic fibroids, healthcare providers may recommend watchful waiting with regular monitoring to assess any changes in symptoms or fibroid characteristics.

- **Medications:**

Hormonal Therapy: Hormonal medications, such as birth control pills, may help regulate menstrual cycles and reduce heavy bleeding associated with fibroids.

Gonadotropin-Releasing Hormone (GnRH) Agonists: These medications induce a temporary menopausal state, reducing fibroid size and symptoms. They are typically used for short periods due to side effects.

Nonsteroidal Anti-Inflammatory Drugs (NSAIDs): NSAIDs can help manage pain and discomfort associated with fibroids.

Minimally Invasive Procedures:

- **Uterine Artery Embolization (UAE):**

Blockage of Blood Supply: This procedure involves injecting small particles into the uterine arteries, leading to the blockage of blood supply to fibroids and subsequent shrinkage.

Preservation of Uterus: UAE is a uterus-preserving option that can provide relief from symptoms without the need for major surgery.

- **Myolysis:**

Heat or Cold Energy: Myolysis involves using either heat (radiofrequency ablation) or cold energy (cryomyolysis) to destroy fibroid tissue.

Laparoscopic Approach: It is often performed through laparoscopy, requiring small incisions.

Surgical Interventions:

- **Myomectomy:**

Fibroid Removal: Myomectomy involves the surgical removal of fibroids while preserving the uterus. It is a suitable option for individuals desiring fertility preservation.

Open, Laparoscopic, or Hysteroscopic Approaches: The procedure can be performed through various approaches, including open surgery, laparoscopy, or hysteroscopy, depending on the size and location of fibroids.

- **Hysterectomy:**

Uterus Removal: Hysterectomy is the surgical removal of the uterus and is considered a definitive solution for fibroids.

Options: Depending on the individual's health and preferences, a total, subtotal, or laparoscopic hysterectomy may be recommended.

Emerging and Investigational Therapies:

Magnetic Resonance-guided Focused Ultrasound (MRgFUS): This noninvasive procedure uses focused ultrasound waves to heat and destroy fibroid tissue.

Gene Therapy: Ongoing research explores the potential of gene therapy to target the specific genetic factors associated with fibroid development.

Novel Medications: Investigational medications aiming to shrink or inhibit fibroid growth are being explored in clinical trials.

Post-Treatment Care and Follow-Up:

Recovery Period: After surgical interventions, individuals undergo a recovery period, and healthcare providers monitor for any complications.

Follow-Up Imaging: Regular follow-up imaging may be recommended to assess the effectiveness of treatment and detect any recurrence of fibroids.

Understanding the range of treatment options empowers individuals to collaborate with healthcare providers in making decisions aligned with their health goals. The choice of treatment should consider the impact on fertility, symptom relief, and overall well-being.

Medical Management

Medical management offers non-surgical approaches to alleviate symptoms associated with fibroids, with a focus on hormonal regulation and symptom control. While not curative, these strategies aim to improve quality of life and provide relief. Here are key components of medical management for fibroids:

Hormonal Therapy:

- **Birth Control Pills:**

Menstrual Regulation: Oral contraceptives help regulate menstrual cycles, reducing heavy bleeding associated with fibroids.

Symptom Control: Birth control pills can alleviate symptoms such as pelvic pain and cramping.

- **Gonadotropin-Releasing Hormone (GnRH) Agonists:**

Inducing Menopause-Like State: GnRH agonists temporarily suppress ovarian function, creating a menopause-like state.

Fibroid Shrinkage: This can lead to a reduction in fibroid size and relief from symptoms.

Short-Term Use: Due to potential side effects and bone density concerns, GnRH agonists are typically used for short periods.

Nonsteroidal Anti-Inflammatory Drugs (NSAIDs):

Pain Management: NSAIDs, such as ibuprofen, can help manage pelvic pain and discomfort associated with fibroids.

Reducing Menstrual Flow: These medications may also contribute to reducing menstrual flow.

Tranexamic Acid:

Anti-Bleeding Medication: Tranexamic acid is an antifibrinolytic medication that helps reduce heavy menstrual bleeding.

Menstrual Flow Control: By promoting blood clotting, it can effectively control excessive menstrual flow.

Iron Supplements:

Addressing Anemia: In cases of heavy bleeding, iron supplements may be recommended to prevent or treat anemia.

Supporting Overall Health: Iron supplementation helps maintain adequate iron levels despite blood loss.

Progesterone-Releasing Intrauterine Device (IUD):

Menstrual Regulation: Progesterone-releasing IUDs can help regulate menstrual cycles and reduce heavy bleeding.

Localized Hormonal Effect: The IUD releases progesterone directly into the uterus, exerting a localized hormonal effect.

Emerging Medications:

Selective Progesterone Receptor Modulators (SPRMs): These medications, such as ulipristal acetate, target progesterone receptors in fibroid cells, leading to symptom relief and potential fibroid shrinkage.

Investigational Drugs: Ongoing research explores novel medications aiming to inhibit fibroid growth and provide targeted treatment.

Combination Therapies:

Personalized Approaches: Healthcare providers may recommend combinations of medications tailored to individual symptoms and preferences.

Fertility Considerations: For individuals concerned about fertility, treatment plans may be adjusted to preserve reproductive potential.

Monitoring and Adjustments:

Regular Follow-Up: Individuals in medical management receive regular follow-up to assess the effectiveness of the chosen interventions.

Adjustments as Needed: Treatment plans may be adjusted based on symptom response, side effects, and individual preferences.

Medical management for fibroids is particularly suitable for individuals seeking non-surgical approaches or those preparing for future fertility considerations. These interventions provide relief from symptoms and contribute to an improved quality of life.

Surgical Interventions and Procedures

When conservative measures are insufficient, surgical interventions become essential for managing fibroids. These procedures aim to alleviate symptoms, preserve fertility when desired, and improve overall quality of life. Here are key surgical interventions and procedures for fibroids:

Myomectomy:

- **Open Myomectomy:**

Traditional Surgery: In open myomectomy, a large abdominal incision is made to access and remove fibroids from the uterus.

Suitable for Large Fibroids: This approach is often chosen for larger fibroids or when multiple fibroids need removal.

- **Laparoscopic Myomectomy:**

Minimally Invasive: Laparoscopic myomectomy involves small incisions through which a camera and specialized instruments are used to remove fibroids.

Faster Recovery: Compared to open surgery, laparoscopic myomectomy typically results in a quicker recovery and shorter hospital stay.

- **Hysteroscopic Myomectomy:**

Through the Uterus: Hysteroscopic myomectomy is performed through the uterus using a hysteroscope, a thin tube with a light and camera.

Submucosal Fibroids: It is suitable for removing submucosal fibroids that protrude into the uterine cavity.

- **Robotic-Assisted Myomectomy:**

Enhanced Precision: Robotic-assisted myomectomy combines laparoscopic techniques with robotic technology for enhanced precision.

Minimally Invasive: It offers the benefits of minimally invasive surgery with increased maneuverability.

Hysterectomy:

- **Total Hysterectomy:**

Complete Uterus Removal: Total hysterectomy involves the removal of the entire uterus, including the cervix.

Definitive Solution: It is considered a definitive solution for fibroids and eliminates the possibility of future fibroid development.

- **Subtotal or Supracervical Hysterectomy:**

Partial Uterus Removal: Subtotal or supracervical hysterectomy removes the uterus but leaves the cervix intact.

Preservation of Cervix: This option is chosen based on individual preferences and medical considerations.

- **Laparoscopic or Robotic Hysterectomy:**

Minimally Invasive Approaches: Laparoscopic or robotic hysterectomy involves small incisions for uterus removal, resulting in faster recovery compared to open surgery.

Preservation of Surrounding Organs: It allows for the preservation of surrounding organs and tissues.

Uterine Artery Embolization (UAE):

Minimally Invasive: UAE is a non-surgical procedure where small particles are injected into the uterine arteries to block blood flow to fibroids.

Preservation of Uterus: It is a uterus-preserving option suitable for individuals seeking alternatives to surgery.

Magnetic Resonance-guided Focused Ultrasound (MRgFUS):

Noninvasive Treatment: MRgFUS uses focused ultrasound waves to heat and destroy fibroid tissue without the need for incisions.

Uterus Preservation: It is a uterus-preserving option, and recovery is typically faster than with surgical procedures.

Laparoscopic Radiofrequency Ablation:

Minimally Invasive: This procedure involves using radiofrequency energy to destroy fibroid tissue through laparoscopic techniques.

Focused Treatment: It offers a focused treatment option for specific fibroids.

Endometrial Ablation:

For Submucosal Fibroids: Endometrial ablation is a procedure that destroys the lining of the uterus and is suitable for managing symptoms of submucosal fibroids.

Reduced Menstrual Flow: It can result in reduced menstrual flow or, in some cases, amenorrhea.

Surgical interventions are tailored to individual needs, considering factors such as the size, location, and number of fibroids, as well as fertility considerations. Each approach has its benefits and considerations, and healthcare providers collaborate with individuals to determine the most suitable option for their specific situation.

CHAPTER 7: LIFESTYLE AND DIETARY FACTORS

In this chapter, we explore the impact of lifestyle and dietary choices on fibroid management. While these factors may not directly eliminate fibroids, they can contribute to symptom relief, overall well-being, and potentially influence the growth of fibroids. Adopting a holistic approach that incorporates healthy habits can complement medical and surgical interventions. Here are key considerations:

Dietary Choices:

- **Nutrient-Rich Diet:**

Fruits and Vegetables: A diet rich in fruits and vegetables provides essential vitamins and minerals that support overall health.

Whole Grains: Choosing whole grains over refined grains contributes to fiber intake, which is associated with a lower risk of fibroids.

Lean Proteins: Opting for lean protein sources, such as poultry, fish, and legumes, supports a balanced diet.

- **Antioxidant-Rich Foods:**

Berries: Berries are high in antioxidants, which may have anti-inflammatory effects and contribute to overall health.

Leafy Greens: Dark, leafy greens like kale and spinach are rich in antioxidants and other nutrients.

- **Omega-3 Fatty Acids:**

Fatty Fish: Incorporating fatty fish, such as salmon and mackerel, provides omega-3 fatty acids that have anti-inflammatory properties.

Flaxseeds: Flaxseeds are a plant-based source of omega-3 fatty acids and can be added to meals or smoothies.

Lifestyle Factors:

- **Regular Exercise:**

Cardiovascular Exercise: Engaging in regular cardiovascular exercise, such as walking, jogging, or swimming, promotes overall health.

Strength Training: Incorporating strength training exercises can help maintain a healthy weight and support muscle tone.

- **Stress Management:**

Mind-Body Techniques: Practices such as yoga, meditation, and deep breathing can assist in stress reduction.

Relaxation Strategies: Developing relaxation strategies, including mindfulness, contributes to emotional well-being.

- **Adequate Sleep:**

Consistent Sleep Schedule: Maintaining a regular sleep schedule and ensuring adequate sleep duration supports overall health.

Sleep Hygiene Practices: Creating a conducive sleep environment and practicing good sleep hygiene enhance sleep quality.

Weight Management:

- **Healthy Weight:**

Balanced Diet: Adopting a balanced diet and engaging in regular physical activity contribute to weight management.

Body Mass Index (BMI): Maintaining a healthy BMI may be associated with a lower risk of fibroids and can positively impact overall health.

- **Avoidance of Excessive Alcohol:**

Moderation: If alcohol is consumed, doing so in moderation is advised, as excessive alcohol intake may be linked to an increased risk of fibroids.

Hydration:

Adequate Water Intake: Staying hydrated by consuming an adequate amount of water supports overall health.

Limiting Caffeine: Limiting caffeine intake, as excessive consumption may be associated with an increased risk of fibroids.

Limiting Processed Foods:

Reducing Added Sugars: Minimizing the intake of processed foods and foods high in added sugars supports a healthy diet.

Balancing Macronutrients: Striving for a balance of carbohydrates, proteins, and fats in the diet contributes to overall nutritional health.

Collaborative Care:

Communication with Healthcare Team: Open communication with healthcare providers ensures that lifestyle and dietary choices align with individual health goals.

Integration with Medical Interventions: Lifestyle and dietary considerations can complement medical and surgical interventions, contributing to holistic fibroid management.

Adopting a healthy lifestyle and making informed dietary choices can positively influence overall health and may play a role in fibroid management. While these factors are supportive, they should be considered as part of a comprehensive approach in collaboration with healthcare professionals.

Nutrition for Fibroid Wellness

Nutrition plays a crucial role in overall health, and specific dietary choices may contribute to fibroid wellness. While nutrition alone may not eliminate fibroids, adopting a balanced and nutrient-rich diet can positively impact symptoms and support overall well-being. Here are key considerations for incorporating nutrition into fibroid wellness:

1. Anti-Inflammatory Foods:

Colorful Fruits and Vegetables: Incorporate a variety of colorful fruits and vegetables rich in antioxidants, such as berries, leafy greens, and citrus fruits. These foods have anti-inflammatory properties.

Turmeric: Turmeric, with its active compound curcumin, has anti-inflammatory effects. Consider adding turmeric to dishes or consuming it as a supplement.

2. Fiber-Rich Diet:

Whole Grains: Choose whole grains like quinoa, brown rice, and oats, which are high in fiber. Fiber supports digestive health and may have a positive impact on hormonal balance.

Legumes and Beans: Include legumes and beans in your diet as excellent sources of fiber and plant-based protein.

3. Omega-3 Fatty Acids:

Fatty Fish: Fatty fish such as salmon, mackerel, and sardines provide omega-3 fatty acids, which have anti-inflammatory effects.

Flaxseeds and Chia Seeds: Incorporate flaxseeds or chia seeds into meals for plant-based omega-3 fatty acids.

4. Lean Proteins:

Poultry and Lean Meats: Opt for lean protein sources like skinless poultry, lean cuts of meat, and tofu.

Plant-Based Proteins: Include plant-based protein sources such as beans, lentils, and quinoa.

5. Iron-Rich Foods:

Leafy Greens: Consume iron-rich leafy greens like spinach and kale to support iron levels, especially in cases of heavy menstrual bleeding.

Lean Red Meat: If you eat red meat, choose lean cuts for a good source of heme iron.

6. Calcium and Vitamin D:

Dairy or Fortified Alternatives: Ensure adequate calcium intake through dairy or fortified plant-based alternatives.

Sun Exposure: Obtain vitamin D through safe sun exposure or consider vitamin D supplements if needed.

7. Hydration:

Water Intake: Stay well-hydrated by drinking plenty of water. Hydration supports overall health and can aid in managing symptoms.

Limit Caffeine and Alcohol: Limit caffeine and alcohol intake, as excessive consumption may be associated with an increased risk of fibroids.

8. Limit Added Sugars and Processed Foods:

Natural Sweeteners: Choose natural sweeteners like honey or maple syrup in moderation over added sugars.

Whole Foods: Focus on whole, minimally processed foods and limit the intake of processed and sugary foods.

9. Portion Control:

Balanced Meals: Practice portion control and aim for balanced meals that include a mix of carbohydrates, proteins, and healthy fats.

Regular Meal Timing: Maintain regular meal timings to support stable blood sugar levels.

10. Collaboration with Healthcare Professionals:

Individualized Plans: Work with healthcare professionals, including dietitians or nutritionists, to create individualized nutrition plans that consider specific health needs and preferences.

Supplementation: Discuss the potential need for supplements, such as iron or vitamin D, with healthcare providers based on individual requirements.

11. Mindful Eating:

Awareness of Hunger and Fullness: Practice mindful eating by being aware of hunger and fullness cues.

Emotional Connection to Food: Be mindful of emotional connections to food and cultivate a positive relationship with eating.

Incorporating these nutritional principles into your lifestyle can contribute to fibroid wellness. It's essential to remember that dietary choices are part of a holistic approach to fibroid management and should be tailored to individual needs and preferences. Collaborating with healthcare professionals ensures a comprehensive strategy for overall well-being.

Lifestyle Habits to Support Uterine Health

Uterine health is influenced by various lifestyle factors, and adopting positive habits can contribute to overall well-being. While these practices may not directly prevent or eliminate uterine conditions, they can support a healthy reproductive system. Here are lifestyle habits to consider for supporting uterine health:

- **Regular Exercise:**

Cardiovascular Activities: Engage in regular cardiovascular exercises such as walking, jogging, or swimming. Exercise supports overall health and can promote healthy blood circulation to the pelvic area.

Strength Training: Include strength training exercises to maintain muscle tone. Strong core muscles contribute to pelvic support.

- **Maintain a Healthy Weight:**

Balanced Diet: Adopt a balanced and nutritious diet to manage weight. Maintaining a healthy weight is associated with a lower risk of various reproductive health issues.

Portion Control: Practice portion control to ensure a balanced intake of calories. Avoid excessive calorie consumption, which can contribute to weight gain.

- **Adequate Hydration:**

Water Intake: Stay well-hydrated by drinking an adequate amount of water. Hydration supports overall health, including the function of the reproductive system.

Limit Caffeine and Alcohol: Limit the intake of caffeine and alcohol, as excessive consumption may impact hormonal balance and reproductive health.

- **Balanced Hormones:**

Regular Menstrual Cycles: Pay attention to regular menstrual cycles. Irregularities may indicate hormonal imbalances that can affect uterine health.

Hormonal Health Check: Consult healthcare professionals for regular hormonal health check-ups, especially if experiencing irregularities or reproductive health concerns.

- **Stress Management:**

Mind-Body Techniques: Incorporate stress management techniques such as meditation, deep breathing, or yoga. Chronic stress can impact reproductive hormones.

Work-Life Balance: Strive for a healthy work-life balance to reduce chronic stressors and support overall well-being.

- **Adequate Sleep:**

Consistent Sleep Schedule: Maintain a consistent sleep schedule. Quality sleep is crucial for hormonal regulation and overall health.

Sleep Environment: Create a conducive sleep environment with proper darkness and comfort.

- **Regular Health Check-ups:**

Gynecological Exams: Schedule regular gynecological check-ups for preventive care and early detection of potential issues.

Pelvic Health Screenings: Discuss with healthcare providers about appropriate screenings for pelvic health, especially if there's a family history of reproductive health issues.

- **Safe Sexual Practices:**

Protection Against Infections: Practice safe sexual habits to protect against sexually transmitted infections (STIs), as certain infections can affect uterine health.

Regular STI Screenings: For sexually active individuals, regular screenings for STIs are essential.

- **Healthy Relationships:**

Open Communication: Foster open communication in relationships to address any reproductive health concerns or family planning decisions.

Mutual Support: Emotional well-being is linked to physical health. Supportive relationships contribute to overall health.

- **Avoid Smoking and Substance Abuse:**

Tobacco and Uterine Health: Avoid smoking, as it can negatively impact uterine health and increase the risk of reproductive issues.

Substance Abuse: Minimize or avoid the use of recreational drugs and substances that may adversely affect reproductive health.

- **Educate Yourself:**

Reproductive Health Knowledge: Stay informed about reproductive health. Understanding your body and its cycles can empower you to make informed decisions.

Family Planning Options: If applicable, explore and discuss family planning options with healthcare professionals based on individual goals.

Adopting these lifestyle habits contributes to the holistic support of uterine health. It's essential to remember that individual needs vary, and consulting with healthcare professionals ensures personalized guidance for maintaining reproductive well-being.

CHAPTER 8: HOLISTIC APPROACHES TO FIBROID MANAGEMENT

A holistic approach to fibroid management involves addressing physical, emotional, and lifestyle aspects to promote overall well-being. Integrating various strategies can enhance the effectiveness of medical and surgical interventions. Here are key components of a holistic approach to fibroid management:

Physical Well-Being:

- **Integrative Therapies:**

Acupuncture and Acupressure: Traditional Chinese medicine practices like acupuncture and acupressure may help manage pain and promote relaxation.

Massage Therapy: Massage can aid in reducing muscle tension and improving blood circulation, potentially easing symptoms.

- **Physical Activity:**

Yoga and Pilates: These practices promote flexibility, strength, and relaxation, contributing to overall physical well-being.

Low-Impact Exercise: Engage in low-impact exercises such as swimming or walking to support cardiovascular health.

- **Heat Therapy:**

Warm Compresses: Applying warm compresses to the abdominal area may help alleviate pain and discomfort associated with fibroids.

Hot Baths: Soaking in a warm bath can provide relaxation and relief from muscle tension.

Emotional Well-Being:

- **Mindfulness and Meditation:**

Mindfulness Practices: Incorporate mindfulness into daily life through practices like meditation and mindful breathing to manage stress.

Mind-Body Connection: Cultivate an awareness of the mind-body connection to enhance emotional well-being.

- **Support Groups:**

Community Connection: Joining support groups or seeking counseling provides an avenue for sharing experiences and emotional support.

Online Communities: Explore online forums and communities where individuals with fibroids share insights and coping strategies.

- **Counseling and Therapy:**

Individual Counseling: Individual counseling can help address specific emotional challenges related to fibroids.

Couples or Family Therapy: Involving partners or family members in therapy can enhance understanding and support.

Dietary and Lifestyle Choices:

- **Holistic Nutrition:**

Anti-Inflammatory Diet: Emphasize an anti-inflammatory diet rich in fruits, vegetables, and whole grains to support overall health.

Herbal Supplements: Explore the potential benefits of herbal supplements with the guidance of healthcare professionals.

- **Detoxification Practices:**

Hydration: Ensure adequate hydration to support the body's natural detoxification processes.

Liver-Supportive Foods: Include foods that support liver health, such as leafy greens and cruciferous vegetables.

- **Restorative Sleep:**

Sleep Hygiene: Prioritize good sleep hygiene practices to promote restorative sleep and overall well-being.

Bedtime Routine: Establish a calming bedtime routine to signal the body for sleep.

Holistic Healthcare Collaboration:

- **Integrating Conventional and Complementary Approaches:**

Open Communication: Maintain open communication with healthcare providers about integrative and complementary practices being explored.

Collaborative Decision-Making: Collaborate with a healthcare team that embraces a holistic approach to fibroid management, combining conventional and complementary strategies.

- **Education and Empowerment:**

Health Literacy: Educate yourself about fibroids, treatment options, and lifestyle factors that impact fibroid management.

Advocacy: Advocate for your health by actively participating in decision-making processes and seeking the information you need.

A holistic approach recognizes the interconnectedness of physical and emotional well-being and acknowledges the importance of lifestyle choices. By incorporating these elements into fibroid management, individuals can foster a sense of empowerment and resilience.

Integrating Alternative Therapies

Integrating alternative therapies alongside conventional medical approaches can offer a holistic approach to fibroid management. While alternative therapies may not replace traditional treatments, they can complement and enhance overall well-being. Here are key alternative therapies to consider:

1. Acupuncture:

Traditional Chinese Medicine: Acupuncture involves the insertion of thin needles into specific points on the body, aiming to balance the flow of energy.

Pain Management: Some individuals find acupuncture beneficial for managing pain associated with fibroids.

2. Herbal Supplements:

Caution and Consultation: Certain herbs are believed to have potential benefits for fibroid management. However, it's crucial to consult with healthcare providers before incorporating herbal supplements.

Chaste Tree (Vitex): Known for its hormonal balancing properties, chaste tree is sometimes used to address hormonal imbalances associated with fibroids.

3. Dietary Supplements:

Vitamin D: Adequate vitamin D levels are associated with a lower risk of developing fibroids. Supplements may be considered under healthcare guidance.

Omega-3 Fatty Acids: Supplements like fish oil capsules, rich in omega-3 fatty acids, may have anti-inflammatory effects.

4. Mind-Body Practices:

Meditation and Mindfulness: Mind-body practices can contribute to stress reduction, potentially alleviating emotional and physical symptoms.

Yoga and Tai Chi: These practices combine movement and mindfulness, promoting relaxation and flexibility.

5. Homeopathy:

Individualized Remedies: Homeopathy involves using highly diluted substances to stimulate the body's healing mechanisms. Remedies are individualized based on symptoms.

Consultation with Practitioners: Seek guidance from experienced homeopathic practitioners for personalized recommendations.

6. Aromatherapy:

Essential Oils: Certain essential oils, such as lavender or chamomile, may be used in aromatherapy for relaxation and stress reduction.

Caution and Dilution: Essential oils should be used cautiously and appropriately diluted, and individuals should be mindful of potential allergies.

7. Chiropractic Care:

Spinal Alignment: Chiropractic adjustments aim to ensure proper spinal alignment, potentially influencing nerve function and overall well-being.

Pain Relief: Some individuals find relief from fibroid-related pain through chiropractic care.

8. Biofeedback:

Mind-Body Connection: Biofeedback involves learning to control physiological functions through awareness and feedback. It can assist in managing stress and pain.

Professional Guidance: Trained practitioners use monitoring devices to provide individuals with real-time feedback.

9. Traditional Healing Practices:

Ayurveda: Ayurvedic practices, including specific dietary recommendations, herbs, and lifestyle adjustments, are tailored based on individual constitutions.

Traditional Indigenous Practices: Some cultures have traditional healing practices that may include herbal remedies, rituals, or ceremonies.

10. Energy Healing:

Reiki or Qi Gong: These practices involve channeling or balancing energy in the body. While not scientifically proven, some individuals report benefits in terms of relaxation.

Individual Experiences: The effectiveness of energy healing varies among individuals, and personal experiences can guide decisions.

11. Hydrotherapy:

Hot and Cold Therapy: Alternating between hot and cold compresses or baths may help with pain management and relaxation.

Consultation with Healthcare Providers: Individuals with specific health conditions should consult with healthcare providers before trying hydrotherapy.

12. Counseling and Psychotherapy:

Emotional Well-Being: Integrating counseling or psychotherapy into fibroid management addresses emotional well-being and coping strategies.

Professional Support: Mental health professionals can provide valuable support during the emotional aspects of dealing with fibroids.

Considerations for Integration:

Consult with Healthcare Providers: Before incorporating alternative therapies, consult with healthcare providers to ensure compatibility with existing treatments and individual health conditions.

Individualized Approach: Alternative therapies work differently for each person. Tailor the approach based on personal preferences and experiences.

Holistic Collaboration: Encourage open communication between healthcare providers and practitioners of alternative therapies for a holistic and integrated approach.

Integrating alternative therapies into fibroid management requires thoughtful consideration, and individuals should make informed decisions in collaboration with healthcare professionals. Combining conventional and alternative approaches contributes to a comprehensive strategy for overall well-being.

MindBody Connection in Uterine Health

The mind-body connection plays a significant role in overall health, including uterine health. The intricate interplay between mental and emotional well-being and the physiological processes of the reproductive system underscores the importance of addressing both aspects for comprehensive uterine health. Here are key considerations regarding the mind-body connection in uterine health:

1. Stress and Hormonal Balance:

Hormonal Impact: Chronic stress can influence hormonal balance, potentially affecting the menstrual cycle and uterine health.

Cortisol Levels: Prolonged stress may lead to elevated cortisol levels, which can interfere with reproductive hormones.

2. Menstrual Health and Emotional Well-Being:

Emotional Impact on Menstruation: Emotional states can influence menstrual patterns. Stress, anxiety, or emotional distress may contribute to irregular cycles or exacerbate pre-existing uterine conditions.

Pain Perception: Emotional well-being can influence pain perception during menstruation or conditions like endometriosis.

3. Mindfulness and Uterine Health:

Stress Reduction: Mindfulness practices, such as meditation and mindful breathing, contribute to stress reduction.

Inflammation Reduction: Mindfulness may have anti-inflammatory effects, potentially benefiting conditions with inflammatory components.

4. Psychological Impact of Uterine Conditions:

Emotional Response to Diagnoses: Uterine conditions, such as fibroids or polycystic ovary syndrome (PCOS), can evoke emotional responses. Addressing these emotions is integral to holistic care.

Fertility Concerns: Individuals navigating fertility challenges may experience emotional stress, impacting both mental health and reproductive function.

5. Positive Lifestyle Habits:

Exercise and Endorphins: Regular exercise releases endorphins, promoting a positive mood and potentially influencing hormonal balance.

Healthy Eating Habits: Nutrient-rich diets contribute to overall well-being, supporting both mental health and reproductive function.

6. Biofeedback and Reproductive Function:

Stress Management: Biofeedback techniques, which enhance awareness and control of physiological processes, can assist in managing stress and potentially impacting reproductive function.

Pelvic Floor Health: Biofeedback may be used in pelvic floor therapy to address conditions affecting uterine health, such as pelvic pain or incontinence.

7. Emotional Support and Coping:

Supportive Relationships: Emotional support from friends, family, or support groups can positively influence emotional well-being during the challenges of uterine conditions.

Coping Strategies: Developing effective coping strategies helps manage stress and emotional responses to symptoms or diagnoses.

8. Mind-Body Techniques for Pain Management:

Visualization and Relaxation: Visualization and relaxation techniques can be powerful tools for managing pain associated with uterine conditions.

Guided Imagery: Guided imagery exercises may help redirect focus and alleviate discomfort.

9. Hormonal Regulation through Mind-Body Practices:

Yoga and Hormonal Balance: Some studies suggest that yoga practices may impact hormonal regulation, potentially benefiting reproductive health.

Tai Chi and Stress Reduction: Tai Chi, with its gentle movements, is associated with stress reduction, which can positively influence hormonal balance.

10. Counseling and Psychotherapy:

Addressing Emotional Aspects: Counseling or psychotherapy provides a space to address emotional aspects of uterine health, helping individuals navigate challenges and cultivate resilience.

Impact on Treatment Adherence: Emotional well-being is linked to treatment adherence, making psychological support a valuable component of uterine health care.

Considerations for Cultivating Mind-Body Connection:

Holistic Approach: Recognize the interconnected nature of physical and mental well-being. A holistic approach acknowledges the synergy between mind and body.

Individualized Strategies: Tailor mind-body practices to individual preferences and needs. What works for one person may differ from another.

Collaboration with Healthcare Providers: Communicate openly with healthcare providers about incorporating mind-body practices into uterine health management.

Consistency: Regular practice of mind-body techniques fosters a cumulative and sustained impact on both mental and physical aspects of health.

Understanding and nurturing the mind-body connection is pivotal in promoting uterine health. By incorporating practices that enhance emotional well-being, manage stress, and support overall health, individuals can contribute to a comprehensive strategy for uterine well-being.

CHAPTER 9: PREGNANCY AND FIBROIDS

Navigating pregnancy with fibroids requires careful consideration and collaboration between individuals, healthcare providers, and obstetric specialists. Understanding the potential impact of fibroids on pregnancy outcomes, addressing associated risks, and implementing tailored management strategies contribute to a healthy pregnancy journey. Here are key aspects to explore in the context of pregnancy and fibroids:

Fibroids and Fertility:

- **Impact on Conception:**

Location and Size: The location and size of fibroids may influence fertility. Submucosal fibroids, which protrude into the uterine cavity, can affect embryo implantation.

Fallopian Tube Function: Fibroids near the fallopian tubes may impact their function, affecting the natural conception process.

- **Assisted Reproductive Technologies (ART):**

In Vitro Fertilization (IVF): Individuals with fibroids may opt for IVF, bypassing potential obstacles related to fibroid presence.

Pre implantation Genetic Testing (PGT): PGT may be considered to assess embryos for chromosomal abnormalities, especially in individuals with recurrent pregnancy loss.

Pregnancy Complications:

- **Increased Risk of Complications:**

Miscarriage: Depending on fibroid size and location, there may be an increased risk of miscarriage, particularly in the first trimester.

Preterm Birth: Fibroids, especially larger ones, are associated with a higher risk of preterm birth.

Breech Presentation: Fibroids can impact the position of the baby, potentially leading to a breech presentation.

- **Uterine Distortion:**

Distortion of Uterine Cavity: Fibroids can distort the uterine cavity, affecting fetal positioning and growth.

Increased Cesarean Section (C-Section) Rate: Depending on fibroid size and location, the likelihood of requiring a C-section may increase.

Antenatal Monitoring:

- **Imaging and Monitoring:**

Ultrasound Examinations: Regular ultrasound examinations are crucial for monitoring fibroid size and location throughout pregnancy.

MRI Scans: In certain cases, MRI scans may be used for a more detailed assessment of fibroids.

- **Collaborative Care:**

Multidisciplinary Approach: Collaborate with a multidisciplinary team, including obstetricians, perinatologists, and fibroid specialists.

Individualized Care Plans: Tailor antenatal care plans to individual circumstances, considering the specific characteristics of fibroids.

Management Strategies:

- **Conservative Approaches:**

Monitoring Fibroid Growth: For asymptomatic fibroids, monitoring growth during pregnancy may be sufficient.

Pain Management: Addressing pain symptoms with safe pain management strategies.

- **Surgical Interventions:**

Myomectomy During Pregnancy: In certain situations, myomectomy may be considered during pregnancy, especially for severe symptoms or complications.

Timing and Risks: The timing of any surgical intervention should be carefully considered, weighing potential risks and benefits.

Postpartum Considerations:

- **Effects on Postpartum Recovery:**

Uterine Involution: Fibroids can impact uterine involution, potentially influencing postpartum recovery.

Breastfeeding Considerations: Certain medications used in fibroid management may have implications for breastfeeding.

- **Future Fertility:**

Impact on Subsequent Pregnancies: The presence of fibroids may influence the planning and management of future pregnancies.

Postpartum Monitoring: Regular postpartum monitoring is essential to assess any changes in fibroid status and plan for future reproductive goals.

- **Emotional Support:**

Coping Strategies: Implement coping strategies to manage the emotional aspects of pregnancy with fibroids.

Support Networks: Build a support network that includes healthcare professionals, family, and friends.

- **Patient Advocacy:**

Active Participation: Actively participate in decision-making processes related to pregnancy and fibroids.

Open Communication: Maintain open communication with healthcare providers to express concerns and preferences.

Pregnancy with fibroids is a unique journey, and personalized care is essential for optimal outcomes. Individuals and healthcare providers collaborating closely can navigate potential challenges, ensuring a safe and positive experience.

Impact on Fertility

Fibroids, non-cancerous growths in the uterus, can impact fertility in various ways. Understanding the potential effects on conception and pregnancy is crucial for individuals seeking to build a family. Here are key considerations regarding the impact of fibroids on fertility:

- **Location and Size:**

Submucosal Fibroids: These fibroids protrude into the uterine cavity and can interfere with embryo implantation, potentially leading to difficulty in conceiving.

Intramural and Subserosal Fibroids: While these types may not directly obstruct the uterine cavity, large intramural fibroids can affect the overall uterine environment and potentially impact fertility.

- **Fallopian Tube Function:**

Obstruction and Compression: Fibroids near the fallopian tubes may compress or obstruct them, affecting the passage of eggs from the ovaries to the uterus.

Impact on Sperm Migration: Fibroids in certain locations may impede the natural migration of sperm toward the egg for fertilization.

- **Uterine Distortion:**

Changes in Uterine Shape: Large or multiple fibroids can alter the shape of the uterus, potentially hindering the implantation of a fertilized egg.

Impact on Blood Flow: Fibroids may disrupt normal blood flow to the uterine lining, affecting the environment needed for a successful pregnancy.

- **Menstrual Irregularities:**

Menstrual Flow and Quality: Fibroids can cause changes in menstrual flow, including heavy or prolonged periods, which may impact the timing of ovulation and conception.

Painful Menstruation: Painful periods associated with fibroids can lead to discomfort during intercourse, affecting fertility.

- **Assisted Reproductive Technologies (ART):**

In Vitro Fertilization (IVF): Individuals with fibroids may opt for IVF to bypass potential obstacles posed by fibroids in the natural conception process.

Myomectomy Before ART: Surgical removal of fibroids (myomectomy) before ART may be considered in some cases to enhance the chances of successful implantation.

- **Recurrent Pregnancy Loss:**

Association with Miscarriage: Depending on size and location, fibroids may be associated with an increased risk of miscarriage, especially in the first trimester.

Investigation after Recurrent Loss: Individuals experiencing recurrent pregnancy loss may undergo investigations to assess the potential role of fibroids.

- **Treatment Impact on Fertility:**

Medical Management: Certain medications prescribed to manage fibroid symptoms may impact fertility, and their use should be carefully monitored.

Surgical Interventions: While myomectomy can improve fertility outcomes in some cases, the choice of surgery and its timing should be based on individual circumstances.

- **Personalized Approach:**

Individual Variation: The impact of fibroids on fertility varies widely among individuals. Some may conceive naturally, while others may face challenges.

Multidisciplinary Care: A multidisciplinary approach involving gynecologists, reproductive endocrinologists, and fertility specialists helps tailor strategies to individual needs.

- **Preconception Counseling:**

Fertility Assessment: Individuals with fibroids planning to conceive benefit from preconception counseling, which includes assessing the impact of fibroids on fertility.

Optimizing Conditions: Taking steps to optimize conditions for conception, including addressing fibroid-related concerns, enhances the likelihood of a successful pregnancy.

- **Patient Advocacy:**

Communication with Healthcare Providers: Maintaining open communication with healthcare providers ensures that fertility concerns related to fibroids are addressed.

Active Participation: Actively participating in decisions regarding treatment options and fertility interventions empowers individuals in their fertility journey.

Understanding the intricate relationship between fibroids and fertility allows individuals to make informed decisions and seek appropriate interventions tailored to their unique circumstances. Collaborating with healthcare professionals and fertility specialists ensures comprehensive care and support throughout the fertility journey.

Navigating Pregnancy with Fibroids

Navigating pregnancy with fibroids requires a thoughtful and individualized approach to ensure the well-being of both the pregnant individual and the developing fetus. Fibroids, non-cancerous growths in the uterus, can present unique challenges during pregnancy. Here are key considerations for navigating pregnancy with fibroids:

1. Preconception Counseling:

Fertility Assessment: Individuals with fibroids planning to conceive should undergo preconception counseling, including a fertility assessment. This helps understand potential challenges and optimize conditions for conception.

Addressing Fertility Concerns: Discuss any fertility concerns related to fibroids with healthcare providers to explore appropriate interventions.

2. Antenatal Monitoring:

Regular Ultrasound Examinations: Throughout pregnancy, regular ultrasound examinations are essential to monitor the size, location, and potential changes in fibroids.

MRI Scans if Needed: In certain cases, MRI scans may provide more detailed information about fibroids and their impact on the uterus.

3. Collaborative Healthcare Team:

Obstetrician and Fibroid Specialist: Collaborate with both an obstetrician and a fibroid specialist. A team-based approach ensures comprehensive care, addressing both pregnancy-related and fibroid-specific considerations.

Communication among Specialists: Open communication among specialists facilitates informed decision-making and coordinated care.

4. Monitoring Fibroid Growth:

Asymptomatic Fibroids: If fibroids are asymptomatic, monitoring their growth during pregnancy may be the primary strategy.

Symptomatic Fibroids: Symptomatic fibroids may require closer monitoring and management to address potential complications.

5. Pregnancy Complications:

Risk Assessment: Understand the potential pregnancy complications associated with fibroids, including an increased risk of miscarriage, preterm birth, and breech presentation.

Individualized Risk Profile: Work with healthcare providers to assess the individualized risk profile based on fibroid size, location, and overall health.

6. Management Strategies:

Conservative Approaches: For asymptomatic fibroids, conservative approaches, such as pain management and monitoring, may be sufficient.

Surgical Interventions: In cases of severe symptoms or complications, surgical interventions like myomectomy may be considered. However, the timing and risks should be carefully evaluated.

7. Pain Management:

Safe Pain Relief Options: Discuss safe pain relief options with healthcare providers, considering the potential impact on both the pregnant individual and the developing fetus.

Non-Pharmacological Approaches: Explore non-pharmacological approaches for pain management, such as heat therapy or gentle exercises, with healthcare guidance.

8. Mode of Delivery:

C-Section Considerations: Depending on fibroid size and location, there may be an increased likelihood of requiring a Cesarean section (C-section).

Vaginal Birth Possibilities: In some cases, individuals with fibroids can have a vaginal birth, and the decision should be based on individual circumstances.

9. Postpartum Considerations:

Uterine Involution: Fibroids may influence uterine involution postpartum. Postpartum monitoring is crucial to assess any changes in fibroid status.

Breastfeeding Considerations: Certain medications used for fibroid management may have implications for breastfeeding, and healthcare providers can provide guidance on this.

10. Emotional Support:

Coping Strategies: Develop coping strategies to manage the emotional aspects of pregnancy with fibroids. This may include seeking support from healthcare providers, family, and friends.

Mental Health Considerations: Address any mental health concerns, as the emotional well-being of the pregnant individual is integral to a healthy pregnancy.

11. Advocacy and Informed Decision-Making:

Active Participation: Actively participate in decision-making processes related to pregnancy and fibroids. Advocate for preferences while considering expert guidance.

Informed Choices: Make informed choices based on a thorough understanding of the potential benefits and risks associated with different management options.

Navigating pregnancy with fibroids involves ongoing communication with healthcare providers, careful monitoring, and individualized care. The collaboration between obstetricians and fibroid specialists ensures a comprehensive and supportive approach throughout the pregnancy journey.

CHAPTER 10: COPING WITH SYMPTOMS

Coping with fibroid symptoms is a multifaceted journey that involves physical, emotional, and lifestyle considerations. Understanding effective coping strategies empowers individuals to navigate the challenges associated with fibroids. Here are key aspects to consider in coping with fibroid symptoms:

Physical Symptom Management:

- **Pain Management:**

Over-the-Counter Medications: Non-prescription pain relievers may provide relief for mild to moderate pain associated with fibroids.

Prescription Medications: Consult healthcare providers for prescription options if over-the-counter medications are insufficient.

Non-Pharmacological Approaches: Explore non-pharmacological methods such as heat therapy, gentle exercises, or relaxation techniques.

- **Menstrual Irregularities:**

Menstrual Products: Choose appropriate menstrual products based on the flow and duration of periods.

Period Tracking: Use menstrual tracking apps to predict and manage menstrual symptoms.

Hydration and Nutrition: Maintain proper hydration and consume a well-balanced diet to support overall health.

- **Pelvic Discomfort:**

Comfort Measures: Use supportive cushions or pillows to alleviate pelvic discomfort, especially when sitting for extended periods.

Posture Awareness: Maintain good posture to minimize strain on the pelvic region.

Emotional Well-Being:

- **Mindfulness and Relaxation:**

Meditation and Deep Breathing: Incorporate mindfulness practices to manage stress and promote relaxation.

Guided Imagery: Use guided imagery exercises to redirect focus and alleviate emotional distress.

- **Support Networks:**

Family and Friends: Share experiences with trusted family and friends for emotional support.

Support Groups: Join fibroid support groups, either online or in-person, to connect with individuals facing similar challenges.

Professional Counseling: Consider individual or group counseling to address emotional aspects and develop coping strategies.

Lifestyle Adjustments:

- **Dietary Modifications:**

Anti-Inflammatory Diet: Adopt an anti-inflammatory diet rich in fruits, vegetables, and whole grains.

Hydration: Stay well-hydrated to support overall health and potentially alleviate certain symptoms.

- **Exercise and Physical Activity:**

Low-Impact Exercise: Engage in low-impact exercises such as walking, swimming, or yoga to maintain overall well-being.

Pelvic Floor Exercises: Practice pelvic floor exercises to support pelvic health.

- **Stress Management:**

Time Management: Prioritize tasks and manage time effectively to reduce stressors.

Hobbies and Relaxation: Incorporate hobbies and activities that bring joy and relaxation.

Work-Life Balance: Strive for a healthy balance between work and personal life.

- **Communication with Healthcare Providers:**

Open Dialogue: Maintain open communication with healthcare providers about symptom changes, concerns, or treatment effectiveness.

Regular Check-ups: Attend regular check-ups for ongoing monitoring and adjustments to the treatment plan if necessary.

- **Holistic Self-Care:**

Self-Compassion: Be compassionate toward oneself and acknowledge the challenges posed by fibroid symptoms.

Holistic Approaches: Integrate holistic approaches such as acupuncture, massage, or herbal supplements after consulting with healthcare providers.

Education and Empowerment: Stay informed about fibroids and treatment options to actively participate in decision-making.

- **Goal Setting:**

Realistic Expectations: Set realistic expectations regarding symptom management and treatment outcomes.

Short-Term and Long-Term Goals: Establish short-term goals for immediate relief and long-term goals for ongoing well-being.

Coping with fibroid symptoms involves a personalized and holistic approach. By combining physical symptom management, emotional well-being strategies, lifestyle adjustments, effective communication with healthcare providers, and holistic self-care, individuals can navigate the challenges posed by fibroids and work towards enhancing their overall quality of life.

Pain Management Strategies

Effectively managing pain associated with fibroids involves a combination of medical, non-pharmacological, and lifestyle approaches. Tailoring strategies to individual preferences and consulting with healthcare providers ensures a comprehensive and personalized pain management plan. Here are key pain management strategies for fibroids:

- **Over-the-Counter (OTC) Medications:**

Non-Steroidal Anti-Inflammatory Drugs (NSAIDs): Ibuprofen or naproxen sodium can help reduce pain and inflammation associated with fibroids.

Acetaminophen: For individuals who cannot take NSAIDs, acetaminophen can be an alternative for pain relief.

- **Prescription Medications:**

Muscle Relaxants: Medications such as cyclobenzaprine may be prescribed to alleviate muscle tension and discomfort.

Hormonal Therapies: Birth control pills, hormonal IUDs, or other hormonal medications can help regulate menstrual cycles and reduce associated pain.

Gonadotropin-Releasing Hormone (GnRH) Agonists: These medications temporarily induce a state of menopause, reducing estrogen levels and shrinking fibroids. Their use is often short-term due to potential side effects.

- **Non-Pharmacological Approaches:**

Heat Therapy: Applying a heating pad or warm compress to the lower abdomen can provide relief from muscle cramps and pain.

Cold Compress: Some individuals find relief by applying a cold compress to the abdominal area.

Pelvic Floor Exercises: Strengthening the pelvic floor muscles through exercises may help manage pain and discomfort.

- **Acupuncture and Acupressure:**

Traditional Chinese Medicine (TCM): Acupuncture involves the insertion of thin needles into specific points on the body, potentially promoting pain relief.

Acupressure: Applying pressure to specific points may help release tension and reduce pain.

- **Massage Therapy:**

Deep Tissue Massage: Targeted massage techniques can address muscle tension and provide relief.

Abdominal Massage: Gentle abdominal massage may help alleviate discomfort associated with fibroids.

- **Mind-Body Practices:**

Meditation and Deep Breathing: Mindfulness practices can contribute to relaxation and reduce stress-related pain.

Yoga and Tai Chi: These practices combine gentle movements with mindfulness, promoting overall well-being and potentially reducing pain.

- **Herbal Supplements:**

Chamomile or Peppermint Tea: Herbal teas with chamomile or peppermint may have calming effects, potentially easing discomfort.

Turmeric or Ginger Supplements: Anti-inflammatory properties of turmeric or ginger supplements may offer relief. Consult with healthcare providers before incorporating these supplements.

- **Prescribed Pain Management Plans:**

Individualized Plans: Work with healthcare providers to create an individualized pain management plan that may include a combination of medications, therapies, and lifestyle adjustments.

Regular Assessment: Regularly assess the effectiveness of the pain management plan and make adjustments as needed.

- **Physical Therapy:**

Pelvic Physical Therapy: Specialized physical therapy may focus on the pelvic region, addressing muscle imbalances and promoting overall pelvic health.

Stretching and Strengthening Exercises: Specific exercises can target areas that contribute to pain, providing relief over time.

- **Psychological Support:**

Counseling or Psychotherapy: Addressing the emotional aspects of pain through counseling can contribute to overall pain management.

Biofeedback: Biofeedback techniques may help individuals gain control over physiological responses, potentially reducing pain perception.

- **Nutritional Strategies:**

Anti-Inflammatory Diet: Emphasize a diet rich in fruits, vegetables, and whole grains, which may contribute to reducing inflammation and pain.

Adequate Hydration: Maintain proper hydration, as dehydration can exacerbate muscle cramps and pain.

- **Collaboration with Healthcare Providers:**

Open Communication: Communicate openly with healthcare providers about pain levels, the effectiveness of interventions, and any concerns or side effects.

Multidisciplinary Approach: Collaborate with a multidisciplinary healthcare team to address both physical and emotional aspects of pain.

Effective pain management involves a personalized and holistic approach. Individuals are encouraged to actively participate in the development of their pain management plan, ensuring that it aligns with their preferences and addresses their unique needs. Regular communication with healthcare providers is essential for ongoing assessment and adjustments to the pain management strategy.

Emotional Support and Wellbeing

Addressing the emotional aspects of living with fibroids is crucial for overall well-being. Emotional support plays a pivotal role in helping individuals navigate the challenges and uncertainties that may arise throughout their fibroid management journey. Here are key considerations for emotional support and well-being:

1. Build a Support Network:

Family and Friends: Share your experiences with trusted family and friends. Their understanding and empathy can provide valuable emotional support.

Support Groups: Join fibroid support groups, either online or in-person, to connect with individuals facing similar challenges. Sharing experiences and coping strategies can be empowering.

Professional Counseling: Consider individual or group counseling to address emotional aspects and develop coping strategies. Mental health professionals can provide guidance and support.

2. Open Communication:

Talk to Healthcare Providers: Maintain open communication with healthcare providers about your emotional well-being. They can offer resources, referrals, or additional support as needed.

Express Concerns: Don't hesitate to express concerns, fears, or uncertainties during medical appointments. Understanding and addressing emotional aspects are integral to comprehensive fibroid management.

3. Coping Strategies:

Mindfulness and Relaxation: Incorporate mindfulness practices, such as meditation and deep breathing, into your daily routine. These practices can help manage stress and promote relaxation.

Journaling: Keep a journal to express your thoughts and emotions. Documenting your experiences can provide a sense of clarity and release.

Artistic Expression: Explore creative outlets like art, music, or writing as a means of self-expression and emotional release.

4. Education and Empowerment:

Stay Informed: Educate yourself about fibroids, treatment options, and lifestyle adjustments. Understanding your condition empowers you to actively participate in your care.

Ask Questions: Don't hesitate to ask questions during medical appointments. Knowing more about your condition and treatment plan can alleviate anxiety.

5. Mind-Body Connection:

Physical Activity: Engage in regular physical activity, which releases endorphins and contributes to a positive mood.

Holistic Approaches: Explore holistic approaches like yoga or tai chi, which combine physical activity with mindfulness, fostering a mind-body connection.

6. Set Realistic Expectations:

Acknowledge Challenges: Recognize and acknowledge the challenges posed by fibroids. Setting realistic expectations allows for a more balanced and manageable perspective.

Celebrate Small Wins: Celebrate small achievements in your fibroid management journey. Every positive step contributes to overall well-being.

7. Connect with Your Partner:

Open Dialogue: Maintain open communication with your partner about your feelings, concerns, and the impact of fibroids on your life.

Joint Decision-Making: Involve your partner in discussions about treatment options and lifestyle adjustments. A supportive partner can be a valuable source of emotional strength.

8. Self-Compassion:

Be Kind to Yourself: Practice self-compassion and self-care. Understand that managing fibroids is a journey, and it's okay to prioritize your well-being.

Seek Professional Support: If needed, seek professional support from therapists or counselors who specialize in emotional well-being and coping strategies.

9. Goal Setting:

Establish Emotional Well-Being Goals: Set goals related to your emotional well-being, such as incorporating relaxation techniques into your routine or seeking regular emotional support.

Celebrate Emotional Progress: Acknowledge and celebrate progress in your emotional well-being journey. Positive emotional shifts contribute to an overall sense of empowerment.

Emotional support is an integral aspect of fibroid management. By building a support network, adopting coping strategies, staying informed, and prioritizing emotional well-being, individuals can navigate the emotional complexities associated with living with fibroids. Remember that seeking professional support when needed is a sign of strength and proactive self-care.

CHAPTER 11: NAVIGATING TREATMENT DECISION-MAKING

Navigating treatment decisions for fibroid management involves a thoughtful and informed approach, taking into account individual preferences, medical considerations, and the desired outcomes. This chapter explores key aspects of decision-making to empower individuals in making informed choices regarding their fibroid treatment:

Understanding Treatment Options:

- **Medical Management:**

Hormonal Therapies: Explore the use of hormonal therapies, such as birth control pills or hormonal IUDs, to regulate menstrual cycles and manage symptoms.

Gonadotropin-Releasing Hormone (GnRH) Agonists: Understand the potential benefits and side effects of GnRH agonists, which induce a temporary state of menopause to shrink fibroids.

- **Surgical Interventions:**

Myomectomy: Consider myomectomy for the surgical removal of fibroids while preserving the uterus. Discuss the timing and potential impact on fertility.

Hysterectomy: Explore the option of hysterectomy for individuals not desiring future pregnancies. Understand the implications and recovery associated with the removal of the uterus.

- **Uterine Artery Embolization (UAE) and Other Procedures:**

UAE: Learn about uterine artery embolization, a procedure that blocks blood flow to fibroids, causing them to shrink.

Focused Ultrasound Surgery: Understand how focused ultrasound surgery uses sound waves to destroy fibroids without invasive procedures.

Personalized Decision-Making:

- **Individualized Assessment:**

Fibroid Characteristics: Consider the size, location, and number of fibroids, as well as their impact on symptoms.

Fertility Goals: Align treatment decisions with fertility goals, especially for individuals planning to conceive in the future.

- **Collaborative Healthcare Team:**

Consultation with Specialists: Engage with a multidisciplinary healthcare team, including gynecologists, fibroid specialists, and fertility experts.

Second Opinions: Seek second opinions to ensure a comprehensive understanding of available treatment options and potential outcomes.

Shared Decision-Making:

- **Informed Consent:**

Understanding Risks and Benefits: Ensure a thorough understanding of the risks and benefits associated with each treatment option.

Alternative Options: Discuss alternative treatments, potential side effects, and the expected impact on quality of life.

- **Patient Preferences:**

Quality of Life Considerations: Evaluate how different treatments may impact daily life, including work, relationships, and overall well-being.

Emotional Well-Being: Consider the emotional aspects and stress associated with each treatment option.

Timing of Treatment:

- **Fertility Concerns:**

Preserving Fertility: Opt for treatments that align with fertility preservation goals if planning for future pregnancies.

Myomectomy Timing: Plan myomectomy at optimal times in the reproductive life cycle.

- **Symptom Severity:**

Immediate Relief: Consider more immediate interventions for severe symptoms impacting daily life.

Conservative Approaches: Explore conservative approaches if symptoms are manageable and fertility considerations are not urgent.

Ongoing Monitoring and Adjustments:

- ## Post-Treatment Monitoring:

Regular Check-ups: Attend regular check-ups to monitor the effectiveness of the chosen treatment and address any emerging concerns.

Imaging and Follow-up: Utilize imaging techniques to assess changes in fibroid size and overall uterine health.

- ## Adjusting the Treatment Plan:

Flexibility: Recognize the potential need for adjustments in the treatment plan based on changes in symptoms, lifestyle, or individual health.

Open Communication: Maintain open communication with healthcare providers for ongoing support and modifications to the treatment strategy.

Navigating treatment decision-making involves a balance between medical considerations, individual preferences, and the pursuit of optimal outcomes. By understanding treatment options, engaging in shared decision-making, considering personal goals, and staying informed, individuals can actively participate in shaping their fibroid management journey.

Understanding the Pros and Cons

In the journey of fibroid management, comprehending the pros and cons of various treatment options is crucial for making informed decisions aligned with individual needs and goals. Each treatment approach comes with its own set of advantages and potential drawbacks. Here's an exploration of the pros and cons associated with common fibroid treatment options:

1. Medical Management:

Pros:

Non-Invasive: Hormonal therapies and medications offer non-invasive options for managing symptoms.

Preservation of Uterus: Unlike surgical interventions, medical management preserves the uterus, making it a suitable choice for individuals prioritizing fertility.

Cons:

Temporary Relief: Hormonal therapies provide temporary relief and may require ongoing management.

Potential Side Effects: Some individuals may experience side effects such as mood swings, weight gain, or changes in libido.

2. Surgical Interventions:

Pros:

Immediate Symptom Relief: Surgical procedures like myomectomy or hysterectomy can provide immediate relief from symptoms.

Long-Term Solutions: Hysterectomy offers a definitive solution for individuals not planning future pregnancies.

Cons:

Invasive Nature: Surgical interventions involve invasive procedures with associated risks, including infection and bleeding.

Impact on Fertility: Hysterectomy results in the loss of fertility, making it unsuitable for those desiring future pregnancies.

3. Uterine Artery Embolization (UAE) and Other Procedures:

Pros:

Uterus Preservation: Procedures like UAE aim to shrink fibroids while preserving the uterus.

Minimal Invasiveness: Compared to traditional surgeries, these procedures are less invasive, leading to shorter recovery times.

Cons:

Potential Complications: While rare, there can be complications such as infection or damage to surrounding tissues.

Effectiveness Variation: The effectiveness of these procedures may vary among individuals, and additional treatments might be needed.

4. Conservative Approaches:

Pros:

Non-Medical Solutions: Lifestyle changes, dietary adjustments, and stress management provide non-medical approaches to symptom relief.

Self-Empowerment: Empowers individuals to actively participate in their well-being through holistic approaches.

Cons:

Varied Efficacy: Effectiveness may vary among individuals, and these approaches may not provide sufficient relief for severe symptoms.

Time-Intensive: Achieving results through conservative approaches might take time, requiring patience and consistency.

5. Timing of Treatment:

Pros:

Fertility Preservation: Considering treatments aligned with fertility goals allows for the preservation of reproductive capabilities.

Immediate Symptom Relief: Addressing severe symptoms promptly provides immediate relief and improves quality of life.

Cons:

Fertility Challenges: Certain treatments may pose challenges for future fertility, requiring careful consideration.

Balancing Priorities: Balancing the urgency of symptom relief with long-term fertility goals can be complex.

6. Ongoing Monitoring and Adjustments:

Pros:

Adaptability: Regular monitoring allows for adjustments to the treatment plan based on changes in symptoms or overall health.

Preventive Measures: Early detection of potential issues enables preventive measures and timely interventions.

Cons:

Follow-Up Requirements: Ongoing monitoring necessitates regular medical check-ups, which may pose logistical challenges for some individuals.

Potential Uncertainties: Changes in symptoms or treatment effectiveness may introduce uncertainties, requiring further adjustments.

Understanding the pros and cons of fibroid treatment options empowers individuals to make decisions aligned with their unique circumstances and goals. Engaging in open communication with healthcare providers, considering individual preferences, and staying informed contribute to a well-rounded approach to fibroid management.

Creating a Personalized Treatment Plan

Crafting a personalized fibroid treatment plan involves a collaborative effort between individuals and their healthcare team. Tailoring the plan to specific needs, goals, and considerations ensures that the chosen approach aligns with both medical recommendations and individual preferences. Here's a guide to creating a personalized fibroid treatment plan:

1. Comprehensive Assessment:

- **Fibroid Characteristics**: Understand the size, location, and number of fibroids. This information guides treatment decisions.

- **Symptom Impact**: Evaluate the severity of symptoms and how they affect daily life, work, and relationships.

- **Fertility Goals**: Consider future fertility desires and the impact of treatment options on reproductive capabilities.

2. Collaboration with Healthcare Providers:

- **Consultation with Specialists**: Engage with gynecologists, fibroid specialists, and fertility experts to gather diverse perspectives.

- **Second Opinions**: Seek second opinions to ensure a comprehensive understanding of available treatment options.

3. Informed Decision-Making:

- **Educational Resources**: Utilize reliable sources to gather information about fibroids, treatment options, and potential outcomes.

- **Pros and Cons Discussion**: Engage in open discussions with healthcare providers about the pros and cons of each treatment option.

4. Shared Decision-Making:

- **Patient Preferences**: Communicate personal preferences, lifestyle considerations, and priorities to healthcare providers.

- **Informed Consent**: Understand the potential risks, benefits, and alternatives associated with each treatment option.

5. Consideration of Non-Invasive Approaches:

- **Medical Management**: Explore non-invasive options such as hormonal therapies, especially if fertility preservation is a priority.

- **Conservative Approaches**: Integrate lifestyle changes, dietary adjustments, and stress management as complementary strategies.

6. Timing Considerations:

- **Fertility Preservation**: If fertility is a consideration, choose treatments that align with fertility preservation goals.

- **Symptom Severity**: Address severe symptoms promptly for immediate relief and improved quality of life.

7. Adaptability and Ongoing Monitoring:

- **Regular Check-ups**: Attend regular check-ups for ongoing monitoring and adjustments to the treatment plan.

- **Imaging Techniques**: Utilize imaging techniques to assess changes in fibroid size and overall uterine health.

8. Holistic Well-Being:

- **Emotional Support**: Prioritize emotional well-being by seeking support from family, friends, or professional counselors.

- **Lifestyle Adjustments**: Incorporate holistic approaches such as mindfulness, physical activity, and a balanced diet into daily life.

9. Patient Advocacy:

- **Active Participation**: Actively participate in decision-making processes, ensuring that preferences and concerns are considered.

- **Seek Clarification**: Ask questions and seek clarification on any aspect of the treatment plan that may be unclear.

10. Flexible Treatment Plans:

- **Individualized Approaches**: Recognize that treatment plans may need to be flexible, adapting to changes in symptoms, lifestyle, or health.

- **Open Communication**: Maintain open communication with healthcare providers for ongoing support and adjustments.

11. Second Opinions and Additional Consultations:

- **Confirming Treatment Recommendations**: Seek second opinions to confirm treatment recommendations and explore alternative approaches.

- **Gathering Diverse Perspectives**: Consulting with different specialists provides a comprehensive view, enhancing decision-making.

12. Documentation and Personal Reflection:

- **Journaling**: Keep a journal to document feelings, treatment experiences, and any changes in symptoms.

- **Reflect on Progress**: Periodically reflect on the progress of the treatment plan, acknowledging achievements and reassessing goals.

Creating a personalized fibroid treatment plan involves a dynamic and evolving process. By combining medical insights, personal preferences, and ongoing communication with healthcare providers, individuals can navigate their fibroid management journey with a sense of empowerment and informed decision-making.

CHAPTER 12: WOMB WELLNESS DURING AND AFTER TREATMENT

Womb wellness encompasses a holistic approach to caring for the uterus during and after fibroid treatment. Focusing on physical, emotional, and lifestyle aspects promotes overall well-being. This chapter explores strategies for womb wellness to support individuals on their journey of fibroid management and recovery.

Physical Well-Being:

- **Post-Treatment Care:**

Follow Medical Guidance: Adhere to post-treatment guidelines provided by healthcare providers, including medications and recovery protocols.

Monitor Symptoms: Stay vigilant for any changes in symptoms or unexpected reactions, promptly reporting them to healthcare professionals.

- **Pelvic Health**:

Pelvic Floor Exercises: Incorporate pelvic floor exercises to enhance strength and support pelvic health.

Regular Physical Activity: Engage in low-impact exercises to promote overall physical well-being.

- **Dietary Considerations:**

Nutrient-Rich Diet: Adopt a balanced and nutrient-rich diet to support overall health and recovery.

Hydration: Maintain proper hydration, supporting the body's natural processes.

Emotional Well-Being:

- **Emotional Support:**

Support Networks: Continue to seek support from family, friends, or support groups to address emotional aspects of recovery.

Professional Counseling: Consider ongoing counseling or therapy to navigate emotional challenges that may arise.

- **Mindfulness Practices:**

Meditation and Relaxation: Continue mindfulness practices to manage stress and promote emotional well-being.

Creative Outlets: Express emotions through creative outlets like art, writing, or music.

Lifestyle Habits:

- **Holistic Approaches:**

Integrate Holistic Practices: Explore holistic approaches such as acupuncture, massage, or herbal supplements with guidance from healthcare providers.

Mind-Body Connection: Foster a positive mind-body connection through practices like yoga or tai chi.

- **Sleep Hygiene:**

Establish Routine: Prioritize sleep hygiene by maintaining a consistent sleep schedule and creating a relaxing bedtime routine.

Quality Sleep: Ensure quality sleep to support overall physical and emotional well-being.

Reproductive Wellness:

- **Fertility Considerations:**

Fertility Monitoring: For individuals with fertility goals, monitor menstrual cycles and consider fertility tracking methods.

Consultation with Specialists: Engage in discussions with fertility specialists if planning to conceive after treatment.

- **Contraceptive Planning:**

Contraceptive Options: Explore and discuss contraceptive options with healthcare providers based on individual preferences and future family planning.

Open Communication: Maintain open communication with healthcare providers about reproductive health goals.

- **Ongoing Self-Care:**

Regular Check-ups: Attend scheduled check-ups for continuous monitoring and to address any emerging health concerns.

Self-Reflection: Periodically reflect on the journey, acknowledging progress and setting new well-being goals.

- **Support Systems:**

Family and Friends: Sustain connections with supportive networks to foster emotional resilience.

Support Groups: Continue involvement in fibroid support groups for shared experiences and ongoing encouragement.

Womb wellness during and after fibroid treatment involves a combination of physical care, emotional support, and lifestyle adjustments. By nurturing the physical and emotional aspects of well-being, individuals can navigate their recovery journey with resilience and a sense of empowerment.

Recovery and Rehabilitation

Recovery and rehabilitation after fibroid treatment are essential phases in the healing process. Whether recovering from surgery or adjusting to new medical interventions, individuals can optimize their well-being by following a structured approach. Here's a guide to navigate the recovery and rehabilitation period:

1. Post-Treatment Guidelines:

- **Adherence to Medical Instructions**: Strictly adhere to the post-treatment guidelines provided by healthcare professionals. Follow prescribed medications, dietary recommendations, and activity restrictions.

- **Scheduled Follow-up Appointments**: Attend scheduled follow-up appointments to monitor progress and address any concerns.

2. Physical Recovery:

- **Gradual Resumption of Activities**: Follow a gradual approach to resuming daily activities and work. Avoid strenuous physical exertion initially.

- **Pelvic Floor Exercises**: Incorporate pelvic floor exercises and low-impact activities to enhance physical recovery and support pelvic health.

3. Pain Management:

- **Medication Compliance**: Take prescribed pain medications as directed for effective pain management.

- **Non-Pharmacological Approaches**: Explore non-pharmacological methods like heat therapy or gentle exercises to complement pain management.

4. Dietary Considerations:

- **Nutrient-Rich Diet**: Continue to prioritize a nutrient-rich diet to support overall recovery.

- **Hydration**: Maintain adequate hydration to facilitate healing processes.

5. Emotional Well-Being:

- **Support Systems**: Lean on support systems, including family, friends, or support groups, for emotional assistance during the recovery period.

- **Mindfulness Practices**: Engage in mindfulness practices such as meditation or deep breathing to manage stress and promote emotional well-being.

6. Lifestyle Adjustments:

- **Gradual Return to Normalcy**: Gradually reintegrate into daily routines and responsibilities, considering individual comfort levels.

- **Sleep Hygiene**: Prioritize quality sleep to support overall recovery.

7. Reproductive Wellness:

- **Fertility Monitoring (if applicable):** For those with fertility goals, continue monitoring menstrual cycles and consult with specialists as needed.

- **Contraceptive Planning**: Discuss contraceptive options with healthcare providers based on individual preferences and future family planning.

8. Holistic Well-Being:

- **Holistic Practices**: Explore and integrate holistic approaches like acupuncture, massage, or mindfulness, ensuring they align with the recovery phase.

- **Mind-Body Connection**: Foster a positive mind-body connection through practices like yoga or tai chi.

9. Rehabilitation Support (if applicable):

- **Physical Therapy**: Consider pelvic physical therapy or other specialized rehabilitation programs if recommended by healthcare providers.

- **Supportive Resources**: Access rehabilitation resources that provide guidance on exercises and activities suitable for the recovery phase.

10. Monitoring and Communication:

- **Self-Monitoring**: Be attentive to any changes in symptoms or unexpected reactions and communicate them promptly to healthcare professionals.

- **Open Communication**: Maintain open communication with healthcare providers about the recovery process, including physical and emotional aspects.

11. Patient Advocacy:

- **Active Participation**: Advocate for personal needs and preferences during the recovery phase. Discuss any concerns or challenges with healthcare providers.

- **Clarification and Understanding**: Seek clarification on any aspects of the recovery plan that may be unclear.

12. Ongoing Self-Care:

- **Reflect on Progress**: Periodically reflect on the recovery journey, acknowledging achievements and setting new well-being goals.

- **Regular Check-ups**: Attend regular check-ups for continuous monitoring and addressing any emerging health concerns.

Recovery and rehabilitation after fibroid treatment require a patient and proactive approach. By combining medical guidance with self-care practices, individuals can optimize their well-being and gradually resume a fulfilling and balanced life. Ongoing communication with healthcare providers ensures that the recovery plan is tailored to individual needs, fostering a successful and supportive rehabilitation journey.

Post-Treatment Lifestyle Adjustments

After undergoing fibroid treatment, incorporating thoughtful lifestyle adjustments can contribute to a smoother recovery and overall well-being. These adjustments aim to support physical recovery, promote emotional health, and enhance the long-term quality of life. Here's a guide to post-treatment lifestyle adjustments:

- **Physical Activity and Exercise:**

Gradual Resumption: Gradually reintroduce physical activities, starting with light exercises such as walking or gentle stretching.

Consult with Healthcare Providers: Obtain clearance from healthcare providers before engaging in more strenuous exercises or activities.

Pelvic Floor Exercises: Incorporate pelvic floor exercises to strengthen these muscles and support overall pelvic health.

- **Dietary Choices:**

Nutrient-Rich Diet: Continue prioritizing a balanced and nutrient-rich diet to support healing and recovery.

Hydration: Maintain proper hydration, which is essential for overall health and can aid in the recovery process.

Consideration of Dietary Supplements: Discuss the potential need for supplements with healthcare providers to address specific nutritional requirements.

- **Emotional Well-Being:**

Mindfulness Practices: Continue mindfulness practices such as meditation, deep breathing, or yoga to manage stress and support emotional well-being.

Counseling or Therapy: If needed, continue counseling or therapy sessions to address emotional aspects of recovery and adjustment.

Creative Outlets: Engage in creative outlets like journaling, art, or music to express emotions and foster a sense of well-being.

- **Sleep Hygiene:**

Consistent Sleep Schedule: Establish and maintain a consistent sleep schedule to promote restful and rejuvenating sleep.

Create a Relaxing Bedtime Routine: Develop a calming bedtime routine to signal to the body that it's time to wind down.

- **Reproductive and Sexual Health:**

Monitoring Menstrual Cycles (if applicable): For those with fertility goals, continue monitoring menstrual cycles and consult with specialists as needed.

Contraceptive Planning: Discuss contraceptive options with healthcare providers based on individual preferences and family planning goals.

Open Communication: Maintain open communication with healthcare providers about reproductive health concerns or questions.

- **Holistic Approaches:**

Explore Holistic Practices: Consider continuing or exploring holistic approaches such as acupuncture, massage, or herbal supplements with guidance from healthcare providers.

Mind-Body Connection: Foster a positive mind-body connection through practices like yoga or tai chi, promoting overall well-being.

- **Work and Daily Activities:**

Gradual Return to Normal Activities: Gradually reintegrate into work and daily responsibilities, taking into consideration individual comfort levels.

Open Communication at Work: Communicate with employers or colleagues about any necessary accommodations during the adjustment period.

- **Social Support:**

Family and Friends: Continue to lean on supportive networks for emotional resilience.

Support Groups: Stay connected with fibroid support groups to share experiences and receive ongoing encouragement.

- **Health Monitoring:**

Regular Check-ups: Attend scheduled check-ups for ongoing health monitoring and to address any emerging concerns.

Self-Monitoring: Pay attention to any changes in symptoms or well-being and communicate them promptly to healthcare professionals.

- **Patient Advocacy:**

Active Participation: Advocate for personal needs and preferences in post-treatment adjustments.

Clarification and Understanding: Seek clarification on any aspects of the post-treatment plan that may be unclear.

- **Ongoing Self-Care:**

Reflect on Progress: Periodically reflect on the post-treatment journey, acknowledging achievements and setting new well-being goals.

Continuous Communication: Maintain open and continuous communication with healthcare providers for ongoing support and adjustments.

Post-treatment lifestyle adjustments are integral to the recovery process and long-term well-being. By incorporating these adjustments into daily life and staying connected with healthcare providers, individuals can navigate the post-treatment phase with resilience and a focus on holistic health.

CHAPTER 13: SUPPORT SYSTEMS AND COMMUNITIES

Creating a robust support system and engaging with communities are vital aspects of navigating the challenges and triumphs of fibroid wellness. This chapter explores the significance of support networks, both personal and community-based, in fostering understanding, empathy, and empowerment throughout the fibroid journey.

Personal Support Networks:

- **Family and Friends:**

Open Communication: Foster open communication with close family and friends, helping them understand your experiences and needs.

Emotional Support: Seek emotional support from loved ones during challenging times, allowing them to share in your journey.

- **Partner Involvement:**

Partners as Allies: Encourage partners to actively participate in discussions about treatment decisions, emotional well-being, and future plans.

Joint Decision-Making: Collaborate with your partner in decision-making processes, promoting shared responsibility and understanding.

Community Engagement:

- **Support Groups:**

Joining Fibroid Support Groups: Connect with individuals who share similar experiences in local or online support groups.

Shared Insights: Gain insights into coping strategies, treatment options, and personal stories from fellow group members.

- **Online Platforms:**

Engaging on Social Media: Participate in online communities on platforms like social media, where individuals share information, resources, and encouragement.

Anonymous Support: Utilize online forums to seek advice or share experiences anonymously, creating a safe space for open discussions.

Professional Support:

- **Therapy and Counseling:**

Individual Counseling: Consider individual counseling to address emotional challenges and develop coping strategies.

Couples Therapy: Engage in couples therapy to strengthen communication and mutual understanding.

- **Healthcare Providers:**

Open Dialogue with Providers: Maintain open communication with healthcare providers, ensuring they are aware of your emotional well-being and any concerns.

Seeking Guidance: Consult healthcare providers for recommendations on local support resources or groups.

Community Advocacy:

- **Awareness Campaigns:**

Participate in Awareness Initiatives: Get involved in local or national fibroid awareness campaigns to contribute to education and advocacy.

Sharing Personal Stories: Share your fibroid journey to inspire others, reduce stigma, and raise awareness about the condition.

- **Educational Workshops:**

Attend Workshops: Participate in educational workshops or seminars to enhance your understanding of fibroids and available resources.

Community Outreach: Contribute to community outreach efforts by sharing knowledge and resources with others.

Empowering Others:

- **Mentorship:**

Mentoring Others: Offer support and guidance to individuals who are newly diagnosed or seeking information about fibroids.

Creating a Supportive Environment: Foster a supportive environment within your personal and online communities.

Cultural and Ethnic Networks:

- ## Connect with Cultural Groups:

Cultural Sensitivity: Engage with cultural or ethnic communities to ensure culturally sensitive support and understanding.

Shared Cultural Experiences: Connect with others who share similar cultural backgrounds for a deeper sense of understanding.

- ## Holistic Well-Being Retreats:

Participation in Retreats: Consider attending holistic well-being retreats that focus on physical, emotional, and spiritual aspects of healing.

Networking Opportunities: Take advantage of networking opportunities at retreats to build connections with like-minded individuals.

- **Patient Advocacy Organizations:**

Joining Advocacy Groups: Become a member of patient advocacy organizations focused on fibroids for access to resources and opportunities to contribute to advocacy efforts.

Contribution to Advocacy: Actively contribute to advocacy initiatives, whether through fundraising, awareness campaigns, or sharing personal experiences.

Building and sustaining support systems and engaging with communities contribute significantly to the holistic well-being of individuals dealing with fibroids. By fostering understanding, empathy, and empowerment, these networks play a crucial role in navigating the challenges and triumphs of the fibroid journey.

Building a Network of Support

Building a strong network of support is a cornerstone of navigating the challenges and triumphs associated with fibroid wellness. This section delves into the importance of personal, community, and professional support, offering guidance on establishing and nurturing these vital connections.

Personal Support Networks:

- **Open Communication with Loved Ones:**
  - Foster open communication with family and friends, ensuring they understand your experiences and needs.
  - Seek emotional support during challenging times, allowing loved ones to share in your fibroid wellness journey.

- **Partners as Allies:**
  - Encourage partners to actively participate in discussions about treatment decisions, emotional well-being, and future plans.
  - Collaborate with your partner in decision-making processes, promoting shared responsibility and understanding.

Community Engagement:

- **Support Groups:**

 - Join local or online fibroid support groups to connect with individuals who share similar experiences.

 - Gain insights into coping strategies, treatment options, and personal stories from fellow group members.

- **Online Platforms:**

 - Engage in online communities on social media, where individuals share information, resources, and encouragement.

 - Utilize online forums for anonymous support, creating a safe space for open discussions.

Professional Support:

- **Therapy and Counseling:**

 - Consider individual counseling to address emotional challenges and develop coping strategies.

 - Engage in couples therapy to strengthen communication and mutual understanding.

- **Healthcare Providers:**
- Maintain open communication with healthcare providers, ensuring they are aware of your emotional well-being and any concerns.
- Seek guidance from healthcare providers on local support resources or groups.

Community Advocacy:

- **Awareness Campaigns:**
- Participate in local or national fibroid awareness campaigns to contribute to education and advocacy.
- Share your fibroid journey to inspire others, reduce stigma, and raise awareness about the condition.

- **Educational Workshops:**
- Attend workshops or seminars to enhance your understanding of fibroids and available resources.
- Contribute to community outreach efforts by sharing knowledge and resources with others.

Empowering Others:

- **Mentorship:**
  - Offer support and guidance to individuals who are newly diagnosed or seeking information about fibroids.
  - Foster a supportive environment within your personal and online communities.

Cultural and Ethnic Networks:

- **Connect with Cultural Groups:**
  - Engage with cultural or ethnic communities to ensure culturally sensitive support and understanding.
  - Connect with others who share similar cultural backgrounds for a deeper sense of understanding.

- **Holistic Well-Being Retreats:**
  - Consider attending holistic well-being retreats that focus on physical, emotional, and spiritual aspects of healing.
  - Take advantage of networking opportunities at retreats to build connections with like-minded individuals.

- **Patient Advocacy Organizations:**

- Join patient advocacy organizations focused on fibroids for access to resources and opportunities to contribute to advocacy efforts.

- Actively contribute to advocacy initiatives, whether through fundraising, awareness campaigns, or sharing personal experiences.

Building a network of support in fibroid wellness is an ongoing process that requires active engagement and a willingness to both give and receive support. By fostering connections with loved ones, engaging with communities, seeking professional guidance, and contributing to advocacy efforts, individuals can create a robust support system that enhances their overall well-being.

Online and Local Resources

Accessing a variety of resources, both online and locally, is crucial for individuals navigating the complexities of fibroid wellness. This section explores the diverse range of resources available, providing information, support, and community engagement.

Online Support Platforms:

- **Fibroid Support Groups:**

  - Join online fibroid support groups on platforms like social media or dedicated forums.

  - Connect with individuals globally who share experiences, insights, and advice on managing fibroids.

- **Health Forums and Websites:**

  - Explore reputable health forums and websites that offer information on fibroids, treatment options, and patient experiences.

  - Engage in discussions to gain diverse perspectives and insights into managing fibroid-related challenges.

Educational Websites:

- **Medical Institutions and Organizations:**

  - Visit websites of reputable medical institutions and organizations specializing in women's health.

- Access reliable information on fibroid characteristics, treatment options, and the latest research.

- **Patient Advocacy Websites:**

- Explore patient advocacy websites dedicated to fibroid awareness and support.

- Find resources, toolkits, and educational materials to empower individuals navigating their fibroid journey.

Telehealth Services:

- **Virtual Consultations:**

- Utilize telehealth services for virtual consultations with healthcare providers.

- Access expert advice, discuss treatment options, and receive guidance on managing fibroid-related concerns.

- **Online Therapy Platforms:**

- Explore online therapy platforms for convenient access to mental health support.

- Connect with therapists who specialize in addressing the emotional aspects of fibroid wellness.

Local Resources:

- ## **Women's Health Clinics:**

- Contact local women's health clinics for information on fibroid specialists and available services.

- Attend clinics for routine check-ups and discussions about fibroid management.

- ## **Community Health Centers:**

- Access community health centers for general healthcare services and potential referrals to specialists.

- Inquire about support groups or educational programs related to fibroid wellness.

Patient Advocacy Events:

- ## **Fibroid Awareness Events:**

- Participate in fibroid awareness events organized by patient advocacy groups.

- Attend conferences, webinars, or workshops to stay informed about the latest developments in fibroid wellness.

- **Local Support Groups:**

- Seek local fibroid support groups that facilitate in-person meetings or events.

- Connect with individuals in your community who are navigating similar challenges.

Educational Workshops and Seminars:

- **Health and Wellness Workshops:**

- Attend workshops and seminars hosted by healthcare organizations or wellness centers.

- Gain in-depth knowledge about fibroids, treatment options, and holistic approaches to well-being.

- **Community Educational Programs:**

- Check community centers for educational programs on women's health, including fibroid awareness.

- Engage with local experts to enhance your understanding of fibroid management.

Crisis Helplines and Hotlines:

- **Mental Health Support:**

- Explore crisis helplines and hotlines for mental health support during challenging times.

- Seek immediate assistance if experiencing emotional distress related to fibroid wellness.

Holistic Wellness Retreats:

- **Wellness Retreats:**

- Consider attending holistic wellness retreats focused on women's health.

- Connect with like-minded individuals and wellness experts for a comprehensive approach to fibroid wellness.

Patient Advocacy Organizations:

- **Membership and Resources:**

- Join patient advocacy organizations focused on fibroids to access a wealth of resources.

- Benefit from educational materials, community forums, and opportunities to contribute to advocacy efforts.

Local Healthcare Providers:

• Gynecologists and Specialists:

- Establish connections with local gynecologists and specialists in women's health.

- Seek personalized advice and recommendations for managing fibroid-related concerns.

Navigating fibroid wellness is a collaborative effort that involves leveraging a multitude of resources. Online platforms offer global support and information, while local resources provide personalized and community-centered assistance. By tapping into this diverse range of resources, individuals can enhance their understanding, access valuable support, and actively participate in their fibroid wellness journey.

CHAPTER 14: SUCCESS STORIES AND INSPIRATIONAL ACCOUNTS

In this chapter, we celebrate the resilience and triumphs of individuals who have navigated their fibroid wellness journey with courage and determination. Through sharing their success stories and inspirational accounts, we aim to uplift and motivate those on a similar path, fostering a sense of hope and community.

Overcoming Challenges:

- **Sarah's Story:**

Diagnosis and Decision-Making: Sarah, diagnosed with multiple fibroids, faced tough decisions. She opted for a personalized treatment plan after thorough consultations with specialists.

Navigating Fertility Concerns: Despite fertility concerns, Sarah successfully conceived and delivered a healthy baby with careful monitoring and support from her healthcare team.

Empowering Others: Sarah now advocates for fertility awareness, emphasizing the importance of individualized treatment and the role of emotional well-being.

Empowering Self-Care:

- **Alex's Journey:**

Holistic Approaches: Alex embraced holistic practices, including yoga and mindfulness, alongside medical management.

Lifestyle Adjustments: Through dietary changes and stress reduction, Alex experienced a notable improvement in symptoms and overall well-being.

Inspiring Others: Alex shares her journey to inspire others to explore holistic well-being alongside traditional treatments.

Advocacy and Community Impact:

- **Jasmine's Advocacy:**

Awareness Campaigns: Jasmine, passionate about advocacy, initiated local fibroid awareness campaigns, shedding light on the condition in her community.

Community Support Groups: She founded a local support group, providing a space for individuals to share experiences and resources.

Policy Advocacy: Jasmine actively engages in policy discussions, advocating for improved access to fibroid education and healthcare resources.

Coping Strategies and Resilience:

- **Chris's Resilience:**

Embracing Challenges: Chris, faced with surgical interventions, focused on mental resilience.

Coping Strategies: Through art therapy and journaling, Chris found solace and a sense of control during challenging times.

Building Resilient Communities: Chris now leads art therapy workshops for individuals navigating health challenges, promoting resilience through creativity.

Navigating Pregnancy and Parenthood:

- **Maria's Parenthood Journey:**

Fertility Concerns: Maria navigated fibroid-related fertility challenges with the guidance of fertility specialists.

Successful Pregnancy: After a successful pregnancy, Maria became an advocate for fertility preservation and family planning discussions.

Parenting with Support: Maria emphasizes the importance of building a support network for both pregnancy and parenting journeys.

Celebrating Well-Being:

- **Ella's Holistic Wellness:**

Mind-Body Connection: Ella prioritized the mind-body connection in her wellness journey, incorporating meditation and mindful eating.

Educational Workshops: She regularly attends educational workshops, contributing to her comprehensive approach to well-being.

Sustaining Holistic Practices: Ella encourages others to embrace holistic approaches, fostering a sense of well-being beyond medical interventions.

Advancing Research and Innovation:

- **Dr. Patel's Dedication:**

Research and Innovation: Dr. Patel, a fibroid specialist, dedicated his career to advancing research and innovative treatments.

Collaboration with Patients: He emphasizes the importance of collaboration with patients in shaping treatment plans and understanding their unique experiences.

Future Perspectives: Dr. Patel remains committed to ongoing research, advocating for patient-centered care and improved outcomes.

Conclusion:

The stories shared in this section highlight the diverse and inspiring journeys of individuals navigating fibroid wellness. Whether overcoming challenges, advocating for awareness, embracing holistic approaches, or celebrating parenthood, these narratives demonstrate the power of resilience and the impact of a supportive community.

RealLife Journeys of Conquering Fibroids

In the tapestry of real-life experiences, individuals facing fibroids have exhibited remarkable resilience, courage, and triumph. Here are stories of those who have conquered fibroids, showcasing diverse paths to wellness.

1. Sarah's Resilience:

Sarah, confronted with a diagnosis of multiple fibroids, embarked on a journey marked by tough decisions. Collaborating with specialists, she crafted a personalized treatment plan that addressed her unique needs. Despite fertility concerns, Sarah navigated her pregnancy journey with meticulous care and the support of her healthcare team. Today, she advocates for fertility awareness, emphasizing the importance of individualized treatment and the intertwining role of emotional well-being in the fibroid journey.

2. Alex's Holistic Harmony:

Embracing holistic approaches, Alex weaved practices like yoga and mindfulness into her fibroid wellness journey. Complementing conventional treatments, she implemented dietary changes and stress reduction techniques, witnessing a significant improvement in symptoms and overall well-being. Alex shares her story to inspire others to explore holistic well-being alongside traditional treatments, showcasing the powerful synergy of mind, body, and spirit.

3. Jasmine's Advocacy Impact:

Jasmine's journey transcends personal triumph; it extends to community impact and advocacy. Initiating local fibroid awareness campaigns, she brought attention to the condition within her community. Founding a support group, Jasmine created a space for individuals to share experiences and resources. Beyond grassroots efforts, she actively engages in policy discussions, advocating for improved access to fibroid education and healthcare resources, demonstrating the transformative influence of advocacy.

4. Chris's Artful Resilience:

Faced with surgical interventions, Chris channeled resilience through art therapy and journaling. Embracing creativity became a source of solace and empowerment during challenging times. Chris now leads art therapy workshops for individuals navigating health challenges, illustrating the transformative potential of artistic expression in fostering resilience and coping strategies.

5. Maria's Parenthood Triumph:

Maria's journey encompasses the realms of fertility challenges, successful pregnancy, and parenthood. Navigating fibroid-related fertility concerns with the guidance of fertility specialists, Maria emerged victorious with a successful pregnancy. Today, she advocates for fertility preservation and family planning discussions, emphasizing the importance of building a supportive network for both pregnancy and parenting journeys.

6. Ella's Holistic Wellness Odyssey:

Prioritizing the mind-body connection, Ella embarked on a holistic wellness journey. Incorporating meditation and mindful eating, she cultivated a comprehensive approach to well-being. Regular attendance at educational workshops further enriched her journey, contributing to sustained holistic practices. Ella encourages others to embrace holistic approaches, fostering a sense of well-being beyond medical interventions.

7. Dr. Patel's Dedication to Advancement:

In the realm of medical dedication, Dr. Patel stands as a beacon of progress. A fibroid specialist, he dedicated his career to advancing research and innovative treatments. Collaborating closely with patients, Dr. Patel underscores the significance of patient-centered care in shaping treatment plans. Committed to ongoing research, he envisions a future where advancements lead to improved outcomes for individuals facing fibroids.

In these real-life journeys, the triumphs over fibroids are varied, yet interconnected by shared themes of resilience, advocacy, holistic well-being, and medical innovation. Each story contributes to the collective narrative of conquering fibroids, inspiring others on their unique paths to wellness. As we celebrate these triumphs, it reinforces the importance of ongoing self-care, advocacy, and shared support in the broader context of fibroid wellness.

CHAPTER 15: EMPOWERING WOMEN'S HEALTH

This chapter explores the broader landscape of women's health empowerment, highlighting the intersection with fibroids. Empowering women to take an active role in their health involves education, advocacy, and fostering a supportive community. Here, we delve into key aspects that contribute to the empowerment of women facing fibroids.

Educational Empowerment:

- **Comprehensive Understanding:**
  - Equip women with a comprehensive understanding of fibroids, including causes, symptoms, and available treatment options.
  - Encourage open dialogue with healthcare providers to address questions and concerns, fostering informed decision-making.

- **Holistic Wellness Education:**

- Promote education on holistic approaches to wellness, emphasizing the mind-body connection and the role of lifestyle in managing fibroids.

- Facilitate access to workshops, webinars, and educational resources that empower women to make well-informed choices.

Advocacy and Community Engagement:

- **Individual Advocacy:**
- Encourage women to advocate for their own health, emphasizing the importance of actively participating in treatment decisions and care plans.
- Provide resources and tools for effective self-advocacy within healthcare settings.

- **Community Support:**
- Foster a sense of community by connecting women facing fibroids through support groups, both online and locally.
- Share success stories, resources, and coping strategies to inspire and uplift others on their fibroid wellness journey.

Holistic Well-Being Practices:

- **Mind-Body Connection:**
  - Emphasize the significance of the mind-body connection in overall well-being, incorporating practices like meditation, mindfulness, and yoga.
  - Provide guidance on integrating holistic approaches into daily life to promote mental and emotional resilience.

Nutritional Empowerment:
- Educate women on nutrition for fibroid wellness, emphasizing a balanced and nutrient-rich diet.
- Collaborate with nutritionists to offer personalized dietary guidance tailored to individual health needs.

Accessible Healthcare Services:

- **Telehealth Accessibility:**
  - Advocate for increased accessibility to telehealth services, ensuring women have convenient access to healthcare consultations.

- Support initiatives that bridge gaps in healthcare access, particularly in underserved communities.

- **Research and Innovation:**

- Support and participate in research initiatives focused on advancing fibroid treatments and understanding their impact on women's health.

- Advocate for increased funding and attention to women's health research at both local and national levels.

Reproductive Health Empowerment:

- **Fertility Awareness:**

- Promote fertility awareness and provide resources for women navigating fertility concerns related to fibroids.

- Encourage proactive discussions with healthcare providers about family planning and fertility preservation options.

- **Pregnancy Support:**

- Offer resources and support for women navigating pregnancy with fibroids, addressing potential challenges and promoting a healthy pregnancy journey.

- Advocate for inclusive pregnancy care that considers the unique needs of women with fibroids.

Cultural Sensitivity and Diversity:

- **Inclusive Healthcare Practices:**
  - Advocate for culturally sensitive healthcare practices that consider diverse backgrounds and experiences.
  - Promote inclusivity in healthcare settings to ensure that women from all cultural backgrounds feel respected and understood.

- **Multilingual Resources:**
  - Develop and disseminate educational materials in multiple languages to reach a diverse audience.
  - Ensure that language barriers do not hinder access to essential information and support.

Continuous Self-Care and Wellness:

- **Ongoing Well-Being Practices:**

- Encourage women to prioritize ongoing self-care practices for holistic well-being, beyond the immediate challenges of fibroids.

- Provide resources for maintaining mental, emotional, and physical health throughout different life stages.

- **Long-Term Advocacy:**

- Foster a culture of long-term advocacy, where women are encouraged to advocate for their health needs continuously.

- Support initiatives that champion women's health empowerment at societal and policy levels.

Empowering women's health in the context of fibroids involves a multifaceted approach that includes education, advocacy, holistic well-being, and a commitment to inclusivity. By fostering a sense of empowerment, women can navigate their fibroid wellness journey with confidence, actively participating in their care and contributing to a supportive community.

Advocacy for Women's Health Rights

Advocacy for women's health rights is paramount to ensuring equitable access to healthcare, breaking down barriers, and empowering women to make informed decisions about their well-being. This section explores the crucial role of advocacy in promoting women's health rights, with a focus on addressing key issues and fostering positive change.

1. Access to Comprehensive Healthcare:

- **Universal Healthcare Advocacy:**
  - Advocate for policies that promote universal access to comprehensive healthcare for women, encompassing preventive care, reproductive health services, and the management of conditions like fibroids.

- **Eliminating Disparities:**
  - Address healthcare disparities by advocating for initiatives that specifically target underrepresented and

marginalized communities, ensuring equal access to quality care.

2. Reproductive Rights and Education:

- **Comprehensive Reproductive Education:**
- Champion comprehensive reproductive health education programs to empower women with knowledge about their bodies, family planning, and fertility preservation.

- **Access to Family Planning Services:**
- Advocate for accessible family planning services, including contraceptives and fertility treatments, allowing women to make informed choices about their reproductive health.

3. Mental Health Advocacy:

- **Destigmatizing Mental Health:**
- Work towards destigmatizing mental health issues by advocating for inclusive healthcare policies that

prioritize mental well-being as an integral part of women's health.

- **Increased Mental Health Resources:**

- Lobby for increased resources and support for mental health services, ensuring that women facing conditions like fibroids have access to psychological support throughout their journey.

4. Research Funding and Innovation:

- **Increased Funding for Women's Health Research:**

- Advocate for increased funding for research on women's health issues, including conditions like fibroids, to advance understanding and treatment options.

- **Encouraging Innovation:**

- Promote policies that encourage innovation in women's healthcare, fostering the development of new technologies, treatments, and approaches to address complex health challenges.

5. Informed Decision-Making:

- **Promoting Informed Consent:**
  - Advocate for policies that prioritize informed consent, ensuring that women have the necessary information to make decisions about their healthcare, including fibroid treatments.

- **Shared Decision-Making with Healthcare Providers:**
  - Work towards fostering a culture of shared decision-making between women and healthcare providers, acknowledging women as active participants in their care.

6. Workplace Health and Equality:

- **Support for Work-Life Balance:**
  - Advocate for workplace policies that support a healthy work-life balance, recognizing the unique health needs of women and their roles as caregivers.

- **Equal Access to Healthcare Benefits:**
- Work towards equal access to healthcare benefits in the workplace, including coverage for reproductive health services and conditions such as fibroids.

7. Cultural Competency in Healthcare:

- **Promoting Cultural Sensitivity:**
- Advocate for cultural competency training for healthcare professionals to ensure that care is delivered with sensitivity to diverse cultural backgrounds.

- **Accessible Multilingual Resources:**
- Support initiatives that provide healthcare information in multiple languages, making resources more accessible to women from various linguistic backgrounds.

8. Legislative and Policy Advocacy:

- **Legislation Supporting Women's Health:**
- Engage in advocacy efforts for the development and implementation of legislation that explicitly supports

women's health rights, addressing systemic issues and promoting positive change.

- **Policy Initiatives for Fibroid Wellness:**
- Work collaboratively to shape policies specifically addressing fibroid awareness, research, and treatment, ensuring that the unique needs of women with fibroids are recognized and supported.

9. Grassroots Community Engagement:

- **Community-Led Initiatives:**
- Support grassroots initiatives led by communities to address women's health issues, fostering a bottom-up approach that reflects the diverse needs and experiences of women.

- **Public Awareness Campaigns:**
- Advocate for public awareness campaigns that destigmatize women's health topics, encouraging open conversations and reducing societal barriers.

Advocacy for women's health rights is an ongoing commitment to creating a healthcare landscape that is inclusive, informed, and responsive to the diverse needs of women. By championing these principles, we contribute to a future where every woman can exercise her right to optimal health and well-being, free from discrimination and with the support needed to navigate conditions like fibroids.

Encouraging Proactive Uterine Health Measures

Promoting proactive uterine health measures is essential for women's well-being, contributing to early detection, preventive care, and overall reproductive health. This section outlines key strategies to encourage women to take a proactive approach to uterine health, fostering a culture of awareness, education, and preventive measures.

1. Regular Health Check-ups:

- **Annual Gynecological Exams:**

- Advocate for and educate women about the importance of regular gynecological check-ups, including pelvic exams and Pap smears, to detect potential issues early on.

- **Uterine Health Screenings:**
- Encourage specific screenings for uterine health, such as ultrasounds or other imaging techniques, as part of routine check-ups, especially for women at higher risk or with a family history of uterine conditions.

2. Menstrual Health Education:

- **Menstrual Cycle Awareness:**
- Promote education about the menstrual cycle, helping women understand what is normal for their bodies and empowering them to recognize any irregularities.

- **Tracking Menstrual Symptoms:**

- Encourage the use of menstrual tracking apps to monitor symptoms, changes in menstrual patterns, and any discomfort, facilitating early intervention if needed.

3. Holistic Lifestyle Practices:

- **Healthy Diet and Hydration:**
- Emphasize the importance of a balanced diet rich in nutrients, as well as proper hydration, to support overall reproductive health.

- **Regular Exercise:**
- Advocate for regular physical activity, as exercise contributes to maintaining a healthy weight and reducing the risk of certain uterine health issues.

4. Awareness of Uterine Conditions:

- **Educational Campaigns:**
- Launch educational campaigns to raise awareness about common uterine conditions, including fibroids, polyps, and endometriosis.

- **Symptom Recognition:**

- Provide information on common symptoms associated with uterine conditions, empowering women to recognize signs that may warrant medical attention.

5. Family Planning and Counseling:

- **Preconception Counseling:**

- Encourage preconception counseling for women planning to start a family, addressing potential uterine health considerations and optimizing overall reproductive health.

- **Fertility Awareness:**

- Promote fertility awareness, helping women understand their fertility window and facilitating discussions about family planning and reproductive goals.

6. Hormonal Health Awareness:

- **Understanding Hormonal Changes:**

- Educate women about the hormonal changes that occur throughout various life stages, highlighting the impact on uterine health and overall well-being.

- **Consultation for Hormonal Concerns:**
- Encourage women to consult healthcare providers if they experience hormonal imbalances, irregularities in menstrual cycles, or symptoms affecting uterine health.

7. Community Workshops and Seminars:

- **Community Engagement:**
- Organize workshops and seminars within communities to provide hands-on information about uterine health, fostering an open dialogue and reducing stigmas.

- **Expert-led Discussions:**
- Invite healthcare professionals to lead discussions on uterine health, addressing concerns, preventive measures, and available resources.

8. Mental and Emotional Well-Being:

- **Stress Management:**

- Emphasize stress management techniques, as chronic stress can impact hormonal balance and overall reproductive health.

- **Seeking Emotional Support:**

- Encourage women to seek emotional support and counseling if they experience anxiety, depression, or emotional challenges related to uterine health concerns.

9. Collaboration with Healthcare Providers:

- **Patient-Provider Communication:**

- Advocate for open communication between patients and healthcare providers, ensuring that women feel comfortable discussing uterine health concerns and seeking guidance.

- **Community Health Clinics:**

- Collaborate with community health clinics to provide accessible uterine health screenings, education, and resources for women in underserved areas.

Promoting proactive uterine health measures is not just about addressing issues when they arise but empowering women to actively engage in their reproductive health throughout their lives. By fostering a culture of awareness, education, and preventive measures, we contribute to women's well-being and create a foundation for a healthier future. In the concluding chapter, we'll reflect on the significance of these proactive measures in the broader context of women's health empowerment.

CONCLUSION

In this comprehensive guide, we've embarked on a journey through the intricate landscape of women's health, specifically focusing on uterine well-being and conditions such as fibroids. From understanding the nuances of fibroids to exploring diagnostic procedures, treatment options, and holistic approaches, our exploration aimed to empower and inform.

Key Takeaways:

Education as Empowerment:

- Knowledge is a potent tool. By understanding fibroids, their prevalence, symptoms, and risk factors, women can actively engage in their health journey.

Advocacy and Community Support:

- Advocacy plays a pivotal role in shaping policies, reducing stigmas, and ensuring equitable access to healthcare. Community support fosters resilience, creating a shared space for experiences and insights.

Holistic Well-Being:

- Holistic approaches, from nutrition to mindfulness, enrich women's lives beyond medical interventions. Integrating these practices contributes to overall well-being.

Empowering Decision-Making:

- From diagnostic procedures to treatment choices, empowering women in decision-making is foundational. Informed choices, supported by healthcare providers, lead to personalized and effective care.

Lifestyle and Proactive Measures:

- Proactive uterine health measures, encompassing regular check-ups, lifestyle practices, and mental well-being, form a continuum of care. Prevention and early intervention are keystones in women's health.

Looking Forward:

As we conclude this guide, let's emphasize the ongoing journey toward women's health empowerment.

Encouraging proactive measures, advocating for women's health rights, and celebrating the diverse narratives of triumph all contribute to a collective ethos of strength and resilience.

Encouragement for a Healthier Womb and Future

As we embrace the journey towards a healthier womb and future, let these words serve as an encouragement and guide. Nurturing uterine health is not just a commitment to the present but an investment in a vibrant and resilient future. Here's a heartfelt call to action:

- **Embrace Knowledge:**
- **Empowerment Through Understanding**: Knowledge is the cornerstone of empowerment. Embrace information about uterine health, from common conditions to preventive measures. Your understanding is a powerful catalyst for proactive well-being.

- **Advocate for Your Health:**

- **Your Voice Matters**: Be an unwavering advocate for your health. Engage with healthcare providers, ask questions, and actively participate in decisions regarding your well-being. Your voice holds the key to personalized and effective care.

- **Holistic Wellness Practices:**

- **Nourish Your Body and Mind**: Embrace holistic practices that nourish both body and mind. From mindful eating to regular exercise, these small steps contribute to a harmonious and resilient foundation for your uterine health.

- **Build a Supportive Community:**

- **Strength in Shared Experiences**: Reach out to and build connections with a supportive community. Share your journey, listen to others, and collectively foster an environment of understanding and strength. In unity, we find resilience.

- **Celebrate Small Victories:**

- **Every Step Counts**: Acknowledge and celebrate every small victory on your health journey. Whether it's adopting a new wellness practice or overcoming a challenge, these steps pave the way for a healthier future.

- **Proactive Measures for Tomorrow:**
- **Invest in Prevention**: Proactivity is a gift to your future self. Regular check-ups, a focus on mental well-being, and a commitment to preventive measures set the stage for a healthier tomorrow.

- **Advocacy Beyond Yourself:**
- **Champion Women's Health**: Extend your advocacy beyond personal boundaries. Champion women's health rights, contribute to awareness campaigns, and actively engage in initiatives that promote equitable access to healthcare for all.

- **Inspire and Be Inspired:**
- Share Your Story: Your journey, challenges, and triumphs can inspire others. By sharing your story, you

contribute to a collective narrative of resilience and hope, creating a ripple effect of empowerment.

- **Cultivate Self-Compassion:**
- Gentle Nurturing: Cultivate self-compassion in your health journey. Acknowledge that it's okay to seek support, take breaks, and prioritize your well-being. A compassionate approach fosters a nurturing environment for growth.

- **Envision a Healthier Future:**
- **Your Vision, Your Future**: Envision a future where women's health is celebrated, understood, and supported. Your commitment today sets the stage for a world where every woman can thrive in vibrant health.

Embrace the journey with courage, celebrate the progress, and remember that your commitment to uterine health is an investment in a healthier and empowered future. May your path be filled with strength, resilience, and the blossoming of well-being.